natural mental health

Also by Carla Wills-Brandon

AM I HUNGRY OR AM I HURTING?

EAT LIKE A LADY: A Guide to Overcoming Bulimia

THE FOURTH STEP: Reevaluating Our Childhood Survival

IS IT LOVE OR IS IT SEX? Why Relationships Don't Work

LEARNING TO SAY NO: Establishing Healthy Boundaries

*WHERE DO I DRAW THE LINE?: How to Get Past Other
People's Problems and Start Living Your Own Life*

*ONE LAST HUG BEFORE I GO: Unlocking the Mystery and
Meaning of Death Bed Visions*

Please visit the Hay House Website at: **hayhouse.com** and
Carla Wills-Brandon's Website at: **carla.willsbrandon.net**

natural mental health

HOW TO TAKE CONTROL

OF YOUR OWN

EMOTIONAL WELL-BEING

CARLA WILLS-BRANDON, Ph.D.

HAY
HOUSE

Hay House, Inc.
Carlsbad, California • Sydney, Australia

Published and distributed in the United States by:

Hay House, Inc., P.O. Box 5100, Carlsbad, CA 92018-5100 • (800) 654-5126
(800) 650-5115 (fax) • www.hayhouse.com

Editorial supervision: Jill Kramer • *Design:* Ashley Parsons

The author of this book does not dispense medical advice or prescribe the use of any technique as a form of treatment for physical or medical problems without the advice of a physician, either directly or indirectly. The intent of the author is only to offer information of a general nature to help you in your quest for emotional and spiritual well-being. In the event you use any of the information in this book for yourself, which is your constitutional right, the author and the publisher assume no responsibility for your actions.

Library of Congress Cataloging-in-Publication Data

Wills-Brandon, Carla.
    Natural mental health : how to take control of your own emotional well-being / by Carla Wills-Brandon.
        p. cm.
    Includes bibliographical references (p.).
    ISBN 1-56170-727-9 (tradepaper)
    1. Mental illness—Alternative treatment. 2. Mental illness—Diet therapy. 3. Mental health. I. Title.

RC480.515.W55 2000
616.89'06—dc21

                                                                00-025650

ISBN 1-56170-727-9

03 02 01 00   4 3 2 1
1st printing, November 2000

Printed in the United States of America

❖ ❖ ❖

*This book is
dedicated to the
three men in my life:
my sons, Aaron and Joshua;
and my partner
for life, Michael.*

❖ ❖ ❖

*T*he *History of Medicine*

2000 B.C.   Here, eat this root.

A.D. 1000   That root is heathen.
                     Here, say this prayer.

A.D. 1850   That prayer is superstition.
                     Here, drink this potion.

A.D. 1940   That potion is snake oil.
                     Here, swallow this pill.

A.D. 1985   That pill is ineffective.
                     Here, take this antibiotic.

2000   That antibiotic doesn't
                     work anymore.
                     Here, eat this root.

(The originator of this is unknown, but its wisdom
is probably not.)

Source: *Vital Signs: Vol. XVII, No. 3, 1998*

Contents

Acknowledgments ix

PART I: UNDERSTANDING SAD AND MAD

Chapter 1:   Emotional Healing the Natural Way 3
Chapter 2:   Depression and Its Companions 17
Chapter 3:   Raging with Anger 33

PART II: HEALING THROUGH RELATIONSHIPS

Chapter 4:   Love Dependency Versus
                 Healthy Self-Love 49
Chapter 5:   Divorce: The End of a Dream 63
Chapter 6:   Let's Talk about Sex 77
Chapter 7:   Abusive Relationships: There Is Hope 91

PART III: DO CONTROL ISSUES CONTROL <u>YOU</u>?

Chapter 8:   Panic Attacks: Secret Protectors 109
Chapter 9:   Sleep Problems and the Fear of
                 Giving Up Control 123

PART IV: REVITALIZING REACTIVE KIDS

Chapter 10: Attention Deficit Disorder:
                 Alternatives to Ritalin 137
Chapter 11: Adolescent Acting-Out:
                 What's It All About? 151

PART V: NO LONGER HIDING FROM LIFE

Chapter 12: Smoking: A Cover for Fear and Anger 167
Chapter 13: Addictive Behavior: Hiding
from Life with Alcohol and Drugs 181

PART VI: LOVING—AND LEAVING—FOOD

Chapter 14: Obsessive-Compulsive Eating 197
Chapter 15: Anorexia: A Slow Death 211
Chapter 16: Bulimia: Running on Empty........................225

PART VII: THE BALANCED WOMAN

Chapter 17: Premenstrual Syndrome:
An Opportunity to Heal 241
Chapter 18: Menopause: It Isn't a Mental Illness 255
Chapter 19: Aging: A Natural Consequence
of Living 271

Afterword: This Is Only the Beginning 287

Appendix I: Healthy Body, Well Mind Diet Plan 289
Appendix II: Supplement for Health 293

Self-Help Resources 297
Suggested Reading 301
About the Author 305

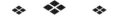

Acknowledgments

No book is ever written by just one person. The birth of any written work involves the creative talent of many remarkable individuals.

Thanks to Dr. Keith Bly and his lovely wife, Amy, for their invaluable computer assistance. Being very computer illiterate, I often run across the street, barefoot and in an absolute state of panic, with a question for Amy or Keith. Both have been very gracious.

The photograph on the back of this book comes courtesy of a very talented photographer. Although studio portraits aren't his cup of tea, Dr. Kevin Katz did a great job of bringing out the best in me.

Jill Kramer, the editor of *Natural Mental Health*, deserves many blessings. Her willingness to take a risk with this project allowed me to put into print what I have been doing in my private practice.

My agent, John White, gets a big hug. For years I have searched for a soul like John, and not so long ago, Higher Powers dropped him in my lap. For all of your nurturing, support, and guidance, much love to you.

I also must express my deepest love and appreciation to my three guys. My boys, Aaron and Josh, have been the guinea pigs for many of the dietary suggestions presented in this book. How often I have heard, "Not another herbal tea mix, Mom," or "What exactly is in this? Are you sure it's edible?" and "Okay, just how awful will this taste?" We have had many laughs over this, and I must say, I admire their courage and love them dearly. If you think my sons were tortured, save some pity for my dear husband of 24 years. The boys have only had to put up with me for a short while. Their father, on the other hand, has had to endure my alternative creations for more than two decades. Thank you, dear, for suffering through the many "tofu" surprises and dreadful-tasting herbal remedies.

Finally, I must acknowledge the clients I have worked with over the years. Many of them came to me in search of alternative solutions to mental health issues. Such a step takes a great deal of bravery. I have learned much from these individuals, and they force me to continue to grow. Many blessings to all of you.

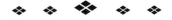

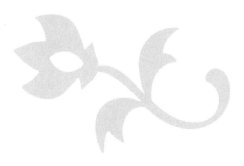

PART I

*U*nderstanding
Sad and Mad

*C*hapter one

EMOTIONAL HEALING THE NATURAL WAY

As usual, it was a great party. Karla, the host of this grand extravaganza, was an expert party organizer. Her parties were always a hit, with never a dull moment. The mood was high, as an old Beatles tune blared out of the backyard speakers. Karla was moving at top speed to make sure that every one of her guests was having a spectacular time. The swimming pool was full of laughing children, splashing away under a light, late-summer sprinkle of rain. Most of the adults had escaped the misty seaside weather by taking refuge under a variety of bright, multi-colored patio umbrellas located around the pool.

As I watched my youngest son bear down on his big brother with a rather large, bright-green water shooter, Karla lightly tapped me on the back and asked, "Have you met my friends over there?" Following her line of sight, I rested my eyes upon a very pretty earth-mother sort of woman, sitting next to an extremely thin, sick-looking man. As I noted the couple with interest, I replied to Karla, "Not yet."

As the evening wore on, I was eventually introduced to this man and woman. While we visited, I noted that underneath his white shirt, the man had a small bag attached to an opening in his abdominal wall. During our conversation, I learned that this poor guy had had several feet of intestine removed from his stomach and that he was gearing up for his second hip replacement surgery. The steroids he was taking to control his ailment had caused premature osteoporosis and brittle bones. Emotionally, he appeared extremely bitter and depressed. While the group continued to talk, I leaned over to Karla and whispered, "Gee, he's only 38, and he's already had several serious major surgeries." I then quietly wondered if he had Crohn's Disease. Being very familiar with this illness, I knew that if I had not taken responsibility for my own healing, this scenario could have been mine.

About 15 years ago, I discovered I was suffering from the aforementioned debilitating condition. After the doctors stuck tubes and scopes up and down every orifice of my body, they withdrew what seemed like gallons of blood from my veins and then pumped my intestines full of a chalky white substance. Then they sat me down and told me that my condition was serious.

Chronic diarrhea, headaches, excruciating spasms, vomiting, depression, exhaustion, and nausea are just a few of the symptoms of the illness. The accompanying depression can be as painful as the physical agony. My choices for treatment were even more depressing. Steroids, the typical mode of traditional treatment, eventually destroys bone tissue, while leaving the sufferer constantly on edge emotionally. Surgery involves removal of damaged, ulcerated sections of the digestive tract. This extreme measure provides only temporary relief, because at the same time, the illness can invade another area of intestine. This leaves scar tissue that can cause a narrowing of the passageway.

The orthodox physicians handling my case recommended the traditional program of treatment. This involved large doses of narcotics along with the strong, toxic steroids. Upon hearing this, I simply felt crushed. One year before, I had checked myself into a drug and alcohol center to cleanse myself of all of the medications I had been taking for this physical condition. After working so hard to "clean up," the thought of returning to that lifestyle pushed me to tears. With much sadness and a deep sense of hopelessness, I gave up personal control. With regard to the steroids, I did what the medical professionals told me to do. Thankfully, something deep inside my soul totally rebelled against the narcotics. Today I'm grateful that I listened to the voice within.

After writing my first book, I went on the lecture circuit. The traveling was exhausting, and the Crohn's Disease was debilitating. The steroids were not helping my condition and were affecting my emotional state. I was constantly irritated, and my mind was racing. To be completely honest, I felt like a real nut case. While in Nashville, Tennessee, for a national conference on Adult Children of Alcoholics, I found the physical and emotional pain of my condition unbearable. It was obvious that the orthodox treatment was not working. I was growing weaker and was feeling extremely sick. I didn't know how I was going to make it through eight hours of lecturing, and jokingly said to my husband, "Well, I guess it's time for me to start making funeral plans. No white lilies, please. I want red roses on my coffin." Although I said this in a joking manner, deep inside I didn't think I would see my 40th birthday.

My time has not run out. I am over 40, and today I can honestly say that I'm physically fit, emotionally at peace, and spiritually alive. My case wasn't hopeless. There were many answers out there, available for the taking. How did this change occur? Quite simply, I decided to take personal responsibility for my own physical, emotional, and spiritual healing. This required becoming directly involved with my own healing process. Passivity was no longer an option.

Over a five-year period, I completely altered my lifestyle and explored a variety of holistic methods of healing. Because the Crohn's Disease had scarred the walls of my intestines, I was not able to absorb the nutrients necessary for maintaining health. In order to rectify this situation, I began to study the digestive tract, vitamin supplements, herbs, and alternative dietary programs.

With the aid of herbs such as slippery elm and aloe vera juice, I was able to begin to heal my poor gut. Eventually, steroids were no longer necessary, but my digestive tract was still weak. I began taking mega-doses of vitamins in a form that provided easy absorption, and immediately my energy began to increase.

Looking at my diet, I knew that major changes were necessary. An alternative health caregiver suggested that I investigate the possibility of food allergies. I discovered that many of the foods I regularly included in my diet were partially responsible for the flaring up of the Crohn's Disease. These food products made healing almost impossible. Today, I abstain from wheat, dairy, and meat products. If I reintroduce these foods into my diet, I can count on relapsing into the disease.

Dealing with the physical body was only the beginning of my healing process. Emotionally, I carried a great deal of anger and was having difficulty releasing it. This locked-up rage also fanned the flames of searing pain in my abdomen. Utilizing acupuncture, acupressure, psychotherapy, and massage therapy, I was able to discharge this emotion from my body. This, in turn, allowed my digestive tract to relax. Exploring traditional Korean martial arts also provided me with an active way to release my anger. And, incorporating herbs such as lemon balm, withania, ginseng, and lavender into my lifestyle helped me cope with the depression that had haunted me most of my adult life.

Once my physical and emotional health began to improve, the voice inside me announced that my spirit was also in need of nourishment. By exposing myself to many alternative forms of spirituality, I discovered a number of heavenly, celestial paths. These included firewalking, yoga, meditation, aura reading, the study of ancient religions, and a host of other traditional and not-so-traditional spiritual experiences. My quest for spiritual nourishment eventually gave meaning to my existence.

One of the most profound messages I received during this transformation validated my initial reason for beginning my venture into holistic health. The message is: "I am responsible for my physical, emotional, and spiritual health," and it is now at the base of all the decisions I make. As a professional caregiver, I try to pass this same message on to all those I serve.

Being a Licensed Marriage and Family Therapist, I am very aware that most of those visiting a psychiatrist, psychologist, or other mental health professional only engage in "talk therapy." In my opinion, talk therapy, by itself, is a waste of time. One might as well flush their money down the toilet. In order for emotional health to take hold, one must be an active participant in the therapeutic process. A psychotropic drug such as an antidepressant, along with a few sessions of talk therapy, can never replace a holistic approach. Recently, I had to explain this concept to a client of mine.

The Holistic Approach Works

Looking at the petite middle-aged woman sitting in my office, I thought to myself, *Healthwise, she really is a mess!* This talented artist, who made a living creating bright, colorful works of art, appeared to be emotionally, physically, and spiritually depleted. Leaking breast implants had poisoned her body. Reading through her "food journal," I saw that, nutritionally, she was starving herself. Depression would be a natural consequence. On top of all of the physical damage, she carried enough unresolved emotional distress for 20 people.

As she searched my face for expressions of approval about her eating habits, she remarked, "I think I eat very healthy foods." Sighing to myself, I wondered how such a bright person could even begin to consider macaroni, doughnuts, bacon sandwiches, and diet soda healthy nourishment for an already toxic body.

She then said, "All I really need is a little pill that will make me feel good, something that will pep me up a bit, lift my mood.

What do you know about antidepressants?"

Shaking my head, I sat down next to her, took her hand in mine, and bluntly said, "There are no quick fixes." Physical, emotional, and spiritual health could be hers only if she would take total responsibility for herself.

For many visiting my office for the first time, the belief is that I will wave some sort of magic wand over them, immediately curing any physical, emotional, and spiritual pain they're experiencing. They look to me to provide quick-fix solutions. When I tell them that their healing will take time, dedication, an attitude of responsibility for themselves, and major lifestyle changes, three-fourths of these suffering men and women never return to my door. Instead, they go in search of the helping professional who will willingly encourage the use of, and even prescribe, the wanted sedative, diet pill, antidepressant, or other traditional medication. Once this temporary "mood fix" proves to be ineffective or fleeting, the emotionally distressed person will go off again in search of another magical resolution.

The current use of medications for mental illness and adjustment difficulties such as obsessive-compulsive disorder, addictions, phobias, trauma, grief, divorce, or other life-cycle crises is at an all-time high. Drug companies are making billions of dollars from the pain of emotionally distressed people. Because they've rejected their own personal power to self-heal in exchange for the care of a physician or psychiatrist, such individuals are easy prey. In our society, we've developed a strong dependence on the medical profession. Thinking, challenging ideas, and responsibility for personal change has been replaced by blind faith in these very fallible human practitioners.

Several months ago, a woman complained to me of a rash. After looking at this angry inflammation, I asked her if she was experiencing any emotional stress. In response, she asked, "What does that have to do with my rash?" I then suggested that her outbreak could be the by-product of an allergic reaction to something in her environment. After pausing for a moment, she said, "You know, this awful itching and burning might be related to a change I made in laundry detergent." Pondering this thought for a minute or so, she suddenly looked me straight in the eye and said, "Also, my sister-in-law has been calling me twice a day, and she's driving me nuts. I could just strangle her!"

Upon hearing this, I said, "Maybe you might want to discharge the anger you have toward your sister-in-law by beating on a stack of pillows or writing an angry letter." I then offered to make up an herbal salve containing clove oil, tea tree oil, chickweed, and calendula for her rash. This particular herbal combination would safely take care of the itch and the redness. I also suggested that she try drinking a cup of skullcap tea or fruit juice with a passion flower tincture when feeling stressed. Both of these herbal remedies have been around for centuries and have the ability to safely relax an overanxious nervous system.

Her immediate response was, "Oh, no, I can't do that! Beat on pillows and take herbs for a rash? No, I must let the doctor decide what it is I need to do. He'll give me a medication for the rash, and he'll probably want to put me on a tranquilizer." Although this intelligent woman holds two Ph.D.'s, when it came to her health, she was unwilling to think for herself.

Like the woman above, too many people have made the medical and psychiatric industry all-powerful. Prozac will not make us whole. Valium will not relieve us of our emotional injuries, and none of the psychotropic medications on the market today will promote spiritual development and self-love. When the newness of the medication wears off, we will once again be confronted with . . . ourselves. Although a few severely ill souls in our society *do* need these medications for their very existence, the majority of us can do very well without them.

In spite of society's conditioning to turn all physical and emotional health matters over to traditional medical caregivers, we must not give up hope. This book is dedicated to those individuals who are willing to accept personal responsibility for their emotional, physical, and spiritual well-being. There is a growing number of people who are investigating how holistic healing methods can work hand-in-hand with Western medicine.

In the area of psychological wellness, the search for more natural methods for attaining a healthy state of mind has begun to take hold. Numerous mental health providers are examining methods of healing that are more in harmony with the body and with nature. Many of us are finally recognizing that total healing cannot happen if a holistic approach is ignored.

Instead of blindly popping an antidepressant for temporary relief from a state of depression, a number of seekers are asking, "What lifestyle changes do I need to make to improve the quality of my life? How can I begin living in harmony not only with my body, but also with my emotions and my spirit? What is available to me for self-healing? Where in nature can I find those tools that will assist me on my quest for a life of well-being and personal responsibility? Are there other steps I can take to improve my emotional state before moving to a pharmaceutical drug and all of its possible side effects?"

Over the years, I have gathered together many natural options for the advancement of mental health. I have incorporated a number of them into my psychological private practice, and the results have been stunning. During the course of my research and studies, I have discovered that there are several safe herbal remedies that can be used to calm a difficult state of mind. Not only is the use of herbs more in harmony with the natural process of the human body, but if used properly, there are few, if any, side effects. It baffles me that such remedies have been pushed aside in favor of often-toxic and dangerous psychotropic medications. A medical path should only be used when all other avenues of healing have failed.

Since the dawn of time, herbal lore has assisted humankind. Every culture can reach back into history and retrieve stories about the village wise woman, shaman, religious leader, or witch who used herbs for the healing of mind, body, and spirit. Our own culture is rich with such lore. Native American Indians thought that herbs not only had great magical power, but that they were also the carriers of spiritual energy. As a result, herbs were honored in ceremonies and rituals, and they were used with great reverence. The purple wild iris or "blue flag" found in the marshy areas of this country was used extensively by Native Americans as a laxative; to increase urination; detoxify the body; and for acne, eczema, and constipation. Understanding that a small amount of this herb could *relieve* vomiting, and that a large amount of the plant would *cause* vomiting, furthered their respect for balance in using nature's remedies.

Mistletoe, a parasitic plant that grows on the branches of trees, was a sacred herb of the Druids. The herb was cut out of the trees by them in a midwinter ceremony and was then passed around to villagers as a common "cure-all" remedy. Mistletoe was seen as an herb with much vitality, and as a result, was viewed as the "semen" of the oak trees in which it grew. Kissing under the sprig of mistletoe hanging over the doorway at Christmastime dates back to this belief. As a fertility charm, the herb was thought to possess magical powers.

According to tradition, those who kiss under the evergreen plant with the sticky berries are also supposed to pick one berry for luck. (The berries are very poisonous and should never be taken internally.) Aside from its charming folklore, the dried leafy twigs of the mistletoe can be used in small amounts in an infusion (steeped tea) to soothe the nervous system, ease anxiety, promote sleep, and relieve panic attacks. Because the Druids understood that not all parts of this plant were safe for internal use, they assisted the population in the appropriate usage of this herb. They were the herbal masters of their communities, and like the Native Americans, they understood the importance of balance in using herbal remedies. Unfortunately, most individuals in our community cannot enjoy the value of this herb because they haven't the knowledge, or because they've been frightened by the risks involved in using this herb improperly. Instead, we turn to toxic medications.

A woman recently telephoned my office in search of a referral to a psychiatrist who would prescribe an antidepressant. I asked, "Why do you think you need this medication?"

In response, she suddenly broke down and shared, "I have three children under the age of four. My house is a mess, and I never seem to be able to get a thing done. My children suffer from earaches constantly, and I'm making monthly trips to the pharmacy to pick up antibiotics for them. These antibiotics put them in a foul mood, and they seem to suffer from a host of side effects. My poor husband is working two jobs, and I'm trying to finish up a college degree. I feel so overwhelmed." After listening to her, I felt exhausted and in need of a large cup of hot ginger tea to reenergize my spirits. I suggested that she make an appointment.

When she showed up for our visit, I immediately recognized that she was using food to nurture herself. After she vented for a bit, I asked her about her eating habits. "I usually snack on the kids' cereals during the day, and then my husband brings home fast food for dinner." Nutritionally, her body was starving and wasn't able to provide her with the energy she needed for a busy life. I then asked her if she and her husband ever had time together away from the children, to relax and be with one another. "Oh, no, there just isn't time." Finally, I encouraged this woman to share her daily routine with me. It quickly became apparent that she didn't have a minute to herself. Emotionally, she was stressed to the edge and lived on a constant merry-go-round of caretaking from sunrise to sunset.

With this information, I was able to offer her a few helpful suggestions. These very simple remedies included a "mother's day out" with her local church group, a regular "date night" with her husband, and involvement in a play group and an exercise class with other mothers and their children. I gave her information on diets for her children to reduce their incidences of ear infections, and recommended that everyone make new, healthy snacking selections from my "Caveman Diet" (see page 100) for those on the go. She could access more relief for herself by taking herbs that can be utilized for effectively increasing energy (including codonopsis, an herb from Chinese medicine used for more vitality); reducing stress (including lemon balm, an herb that safely eases physical tension); and easing symptoms of premenstrual syndrome (with agnus-castus, an herb that has been researched in the United Kingdom and Germany for over 30 years for its specific hormonal effect on the body). By simply improving her own diet, implementing the suggested lifestyle changes, and encouraging the daily use of certain herbs, this woman's emotional distress began to lessen.

If the body is starving nutritionally, this will impact one's mood, decision-making processes, and sense of well-being. Diet is directly related to our emotional health. Sadly, this issue is rarely addressed by the traditional mental health provider. Most of us are unaware that Vitamin B1, found in broccoli, avocado, almonds, raisins, and rice, is useful in combating stress; or that Vitamin B12, found in beans, grains, nuts, and garlic, helps maintain a healthy nervous system. These are just 2 of 22 vitamins necessary for maintaining a healthy emotional and physical state. The majority of the population believes that the mineral calcium is only necessary for strong bones and teeth. Most of us are unaware that it also contributes to a positive state of mind. Calcium, which is found in dairy products, carrots, figs, sunflower seeds, oranges, lentils, and oats, is just one of 20 minerals that help support physical and mental health. Vitamins and minerals can be found in whole foods, herbs, and nutritional supplements.

Lifestyle can also have a huge impact on our emotional state. Current lifestyle situations can leave us feeling depressed, prone to rage, hopeless, alone, afraid, overwhelmed, and even suicidal. An inability to effectively deal with stress, poor time-management skills, excessive alcohol or drug use, unhealthy relationships, communication difficulties, excessive work schedules (on the job and at home), limited leisure time, unresolved issues involving spiritual questions, and more can greatly contribute to feelings of dissatisfaction. This, in turn, can affect our emotional, physical, and spiritual wellness.

Mental health is also dependent on the resolution of unresolved trauma. The trauma might involve a troubled childhood, a lost love affair, a divorce, the death of a loved one, a major job change or geographical move, caring for aging parents, difficulty in raising children, a sexual assault, or any other number of intense life experiences. Mentally pushing these experiences aside does not relieve one of the emotions. Eventually these emotions will surface again and again in the form of depression, rage, addictions, and a host of other symptoms. Simple psychological exercises can begin to address these issues.

Those suffering from emotional pain can begin to mend themselves with active psychological healing techniques, healthy lifestyle changes, nutrition, and herbalism. Utilizing this holistic approach can have many long-term benefits. *Natural Mental Health* will provide you with holistic solutions to mental health issues such as attention deficit disorder

(ADD), addictions, sleep difficulties, panic attacks, sexual trauma, rage attacks, and more.

The following chapters take one emotional difficulty at a time and present a three-part healing process for that mental state. At the beginning of each chapter, the emotional issue will be described. Symptoms will be addressed, and likely causes will be presented. Techniques for addressing these psychological problems will be offered. Next, lifestyle issues will be discussed. The importance of stress levels, sleep, exercise, emotional support from others, therapy, and other healthy life factors will also be explored. Third, nutrition will be discussed, as dietary issues often play a powerful role in how we function emotionally. In that section, the use of certain herbs will be suggested.

Since my basic message is "You are your best healer," I will encourage you to become your own herbalist and to take up the study of herbs. Today the public can buy herbs over-the-counter from health-food stores and even drugstores, but using them does require a responsible attitude. Before using any herb, always educate yourself on its properties. And, realize that although one herb may work for one particular person, it may be ineffective for another. It's always important to understand that herbs are not to be taken lightly. Some herbs, if taken inappropriately or with traditional pharmaceutical medications, can have devastating effects on the human body. In certain situations, a particular physical disorder may preclude a person from ingesting a particular herb or vitamin. If you aren't sure about a suggested herb or nutritional supplement, research it for yourself. For your education, I have provided a number of excellent books on herbs, vitamins, and more in the "Suggested Reading" section of this book.

It's my deepest desire that *Natural Mental Health* will encourage you to take a more active role in your physical and emotional life. This type of action not only heals the body and mind, but it also heals the spirit. When we start to accept responsibility for our emotional health, this action, in turn, spills over into family relationships and community involvement, and heightens environmental awareness.

Although the thought of self-responsibility may be frightening, I still strongly believe that you're ready to walk through this fear. If you weren't ready, you never would have picked up this book. You deserve to feel empowered with the knowledge that everything you need for complete health resides within you. You don't have to give up your power to a toxic drug. Remember, such drugs are a last resort. Begin to trust yourself, and listen to that small voice from within that says, "You can do it." I did, and it worked.

My best to you as you begin your own journey of personal healing.

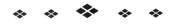

Chapter two

DEPRESSION AND ITS COMPANIONS

For Marianne, life seemed very bleak. There was an emptiness lodged deep within her spirit. While dragging her tired body out of bed, she thought, *My existence seems totally pointless.* She had spent another sleepless night tossing and turning. After putting on her old bathrobe, Marianne made her way to the kitchen

In the hallway, she heard her two yellow lovebirds madly arguing with each other. At one time, such "bird bickering" would have brought a smile to her face. But not this morning. For the last several months, joy was nowhere to be found. Instead, a grievous sense of sadness penetrated every cell of her being. Tightening her robe around her waist, Marianne looked at her birds and said, "Happiness, truly, is just a distant memory."

Once in the kitchen, Marianne groaned, "I just don't have the energy to deal with this." Looking at the sink, she saw the dirty blue-flowered dishes from last night's Chinese take-out meal stacked haphazardly alongside this morning's breakfast plates, cups, and saucers. Shaking her head in dismay, she cried, "Just because the kids are leaving for college next month doesn't mean they no longer have to pick up after themselves. I wish someone would help me with this house. Where is my husband when I need him?" After pouring herself a cup of coffee, she dumped some artificial sweetener into the dark brew and thought, *Maybe this will perk me up.*

After several cups of coffee, Marianne's mood had not improved. She knew it was time to pull herself together for work, but for some reason, she just couldn't force her body to rise out of her chair. "I just detest my job. I think I'll call in sick today." Puff, her big orange-and-brown tabby cat, jumped up on her lap. After kneading her yellow, fuzzy bathrobe with his paws, he settled down for a nap. Looking at him, she wondered, *How can he be so happy?* With this, her tears began to flow. Hugging her purring tabby, Marianne began to weep uncontrollably.

"How much longer will I be in this black hole?"

Every now and then, we all experience depression. The loss of a loved one, job difficulties, a painful divorce, children leaving home, an illness, financial difficulties, a failed love affair, a move, and a variety of other life changes can produce a temporary sense of despair. If addressed, these dark moods eventually depart. If ignored, such an emotional state can turn into a serious clinical depression.

Childhood abuse, a messy parental divorce, a rape, early death of a parent or sibling, and other unresolved traumatic issues can perpetuate lifelong depression. Such a frame of mind can often set the stage for self-medication with food misuse, alcohol, excessive sexual acting-out, illegal drug use, or *legal* drug misuse. Depressive states can also be accompanied by weight gains or losses, extreme fatigue, excessive hopelessness, low sex drive, sleep difficulties, digestive disorders, teeth grinding, colds, low self-esteem, and listlessness.

Traditional treatment usually involves a few talk-therapy sessions and a prescription for an antidepressant. Because such medications can have harsh side effects, I strongly suggest that

Depression and Its Companions

they only be used as a last resort. A holistic approach to addressing this disorder should always be implemented before turning to such drugs.

The Psychology of Depression

— **Unresolved grief.** When depression is relentless and constant, chances are that it has one of two origins—unresolved feelings or physical difficulties. Often, the two go hand-in-hand. Let's begin by taking a look at the emotional side of depression. Grief that has built up over a number of years can produce a clinical depression. Using Marianne as our example of a clinically depressed person, let's examine more closely those situations contributing to her emotional state.

Marianne has several grief issues to contend with. Her marriage is less than satisfactory, and her husband has been pulling away from her for some time and she doesn't know how to resolve this problem. Initially she was angry with him, but now this emotion has turned into despair. Unexpressed anger will eventually turn inward, into depression.

Next, Marianne's children are getting ready to leave for college. Her life has rotated around her girls, and without them, she doesn't know what she'll do. This, too, is a grief issue. At the bottom of many depressive states is unexpressed sadness over a loss.

In addition, Marianne doesn't like her job and she feels unappreciated. She's beginning to feel as though the hours spent at her job are a waste of her time, but she doesn't know what to do about it. A sense of powerless and hopelessness can contribute to depression, too.

To compound these situations, a year ago her mother passed away. Marianne cried several times at the funeral, but after that, the feelings of grief were too great to bear, so she shut them down.

All of the above emotionally triggering issues have finally

caught up with this woman, and she is overwhelmed with depression. Poor Marianne doesn't know where to begin to get help.

Your depression could also be the by-product of a number of unresolved life losses and disappointments. A good exercise is to get out a piece of paper and write down all of these disappointments and losses you've experienced over the last five years. Yes, your list might be long, but that's all right. Next, write a letter to your concept of God, a Higher Power, angels, or guides about these issues. When you've finished your letter, read it to a therapist, spiritual advisor, or health caregiver. Notice how you feel as you go through your letter. Those issues that trigger strong emotions for you just might be at the core of your depression.

— **Stuffed emotions.** As noted, clinical depression can be the by-product of intense feelings related to unresolved grief issues. If we do not feel all of our emotions as they surface, they can eventually accumulate into one large, dark depression.

When it comes to grief, most of us are like Marianne. We don't know what to do with our tears and are frightened of our anger. After repressing these feelings over and over again, often for a period of years, we can find ourselves haunted by a seemingly inexplicable depression. After you've completed the first step in healing (composing your list of disappointments and the letter to your Higher Power) and have read your letter out loud, you will quickly realize which losses and disappointments are still emotionally overwhelming for you. Don't stuff these feelings away. Feel the grief, pain, and sorrow. Cry as long as you need to. Express your anger and rage. Scream and yell at the top of your lungs. By releasing these emotions, you will begin to break up the depression. If you're unable to process these feelings on your own, get some professional help.

— **Visit your health-care provider.** As mentioned earlier, our physical health can contribute to depression. At times, depression can be compounded by physical problems involving hormones, a long illness, blood-sugar disorders, alcohol, drug or food addictions, heart attack or heart surgery, and a host of other physical conditions. To determine whether or not physical issues are contributing to your depression, it's important for you to get a thorough physical from your health-care provider. The kind words of a nurturing, reassuring health-care practitioner can do a world of good.

Addressing the emotional, and possibly physical, origins of your depressive state of mind is essential. In addition, your healing can be greatly enhanced with a number of lifestyle changes.

Lifestyle Remedies for Depression

— **Get a routine going.** When we're depressed, life just feels difficult. Everyday tasks seem impossible, so developing a daily routine and sticking to it will give an emotionally disordered life an anchor.

Begin by arising at the same time each day. Once you're awake, try to get out of bed as soon as possible. Move your body and get those endorphins pumping. Endorphins are chemicals that can counter depression. Physical activity helps the body produce endorphins. Make your bed, take a brisk shower, walk the dog, have a yoga session, or climb up and down the stairs. While you're climbing those stairs or riding that bike, cry, scream, and curse about how hard it is to get moving. If you can't motivate yourself, ask your partner, a family member, or friend to come over and cheer you on.

Take a piece of paper and write out a daily schedule that includes everyday tasks such as taking the kids to school, going to the grocery store, brushing your teeth, eating meals, renting videos, working at the office, and so on. Then rigidly follow this schedule. If you can accomplish your "daily living tasks," this will lift your mood and increase your self-esteem.

— **Speaking of self-esteem.** When was the last time you nurtured yourself with a massage? Massages are great for releasing pent-up emotions. Years ago I was severely depressed and couldn't figure out why. To remedy the problem, I committed myself to visiting a massage therapist for six weeks. After just two sessions, grief about the death of my mother surfaced. At that time, she had been dead for 15 years, but I had never fully recovered from this loss. Interestingly, my depression had set in on the day of her death anniversary. Not only can a massage connect you with those feelings that your depression may be covering, but it can improve your self-esteem about your body. When you nurture your body with gentle touch, you are loving yourself, and this enhances your self-image.

— **Explore your creativity and spirituality.** Believe it or not, we tend to make our greatest spiritual strides when we're in the depths of despair. How can you accomplish this type of growth? Well, by forcing yourself to return to creative hobbies such as dancing, painting, music, sculpting, or any other creative endeavor, you'll be nurturing your spiritual side.

During this time, it will also be important for you to examine your spiritual beliefs to see if you're angry at God, your Higher Power, your angels, or your guides. Feeling cast aside by God or someone you love and trust, can create depression. Underneath this dark mood often lies a great deal of anger. If you feel you have issues of abandonment with God or a loved one, try the following exercise:

Close your eyes and visualize your concept of God or your loved one. Share with them how alone you feel. As you do this imagery work, cry and express your pain. Next, visualize yourself becoming rageful about this sense of rejection or abandonment. Imagine yourself telling God how this feels. After you've done this imagery work, continue to heal your loneliness, hurt, and rage with a ritual or prayer, through artistic expression, or in meditation.

By the way, the death of a loved one often feels like abandonment. It was important for me to go to my mother's grave to tell her how abandoned I'd felt when she passed. I also had to own my anger with God. As a young woman, I was furious with God for taking her away. I then carried these feelings of abandonment, grief, and rage into adulthood. These unexpressed feelings eventually manifested in adulthood as a serious depression. Today, I no longer believe that my mother's early death was God's fault.

— **Self-talk.** Many of us carry messages from the past with us. I'm six feet tall and have size-12 feet. During my youth, I was made fun of by both family members and friends. As an adult, I continued to pound myself with negative childhood messages, especially if I were feeling depressed: *Oh, you're just a big, ugly oaf! Stop acting like such a freak!* Other negative statements I used to beat myself up with included phrases such as: *You're just plain lazy* (or *fat* or *disgusting*). *Are you crazy? Stop acting so stupid, pathetic, dramatic, dumb, ignorant, childish.* And so on. These messages can follow us into adulthood. How do you talk to yourself when you're feeling blue or have made a mistake? Sit down and make a list of all of the negative messages you heard as a child and adolescent.

As an example, for years, whenever I made a mistake, I called myself *dummy*. This word didn't exactly help my self-esteem. When I realized what I was doing, it was necessary for me to delete "dummy" from my vocabulary and replace it with statements such as: *It's okay for me to make a mistake. I have a right to exist. I am lovable. Life is full of valuable lessons for me to learn. I am a bright, creative woman.*

After you've made your list of negative self-talk messages, make sure you replace them with positive affirmations such as the ones I've listed above.

— Look at your environment. Are you dressing in black, keeping your blinds closed, and listening to depressing music? If you are, *stop it.* We unconsciously slip into certain behaviors when we're feeling down. Let's take a look at how our environment impacts our mood.

Dark colors will perpetuate a "blue mood," so open your windows and let the sun flood your living space. A lack of sunlight has been linked to depression, so stay out of dark rooms. Dark-colored clothes also keep us bogged down emotionally.

According to the ancient Chinese art of Feng Shui, your living environment directly impacts your emotional and physical well-being. Color plays a big part in Feng Shui. When I'm feeling extremely depressed, I just have to surround myself with the color green. Several years ago, I learned that according to Feng Shui tradition, green is a wonderful color for relieving depression. Investigate books on color therapy and Feng Shui to determine which colors will work for you.

Finally, music has a powerful influence on how we feel. If you're having trouble breaking up a depressive state of mind, turn on some classical, Celtic, or New Age music. Certain musical pieces can assist us in discharging sadness or anger, lifting our spirits, or in healing a broken heart. Find out what works for you.

When we're depressed, we must attend to our lifestyle and psychological needs. In addition, we must take care of our nutritional requirements. When depressed, we tend to forget to make note of what we're putting in our body. Fast, greasy foods replace healthy proteins; and sugary snacks leave little room for fruits, fiber, and vegetables. Foods absolutely affect our moods. For example, junk food contributes to a melancholy mind-set. Nurturing ourselves with healthy foods, vitamins, minerals, and herbs will lift the darkness of a black mood.

Nutrition and Herbs for Alleviating Depression

—**A balanced diet.** Now is not the time to try the latest tabloid or celebrity-endorsed diet. A menu rich in complex carbohydrates will increase your serotonin production. Serotonin is a neurotransmitter that helps carry nerve impulses in the brain from one nerve cell to the next. Low serotonin has been linked to depressive emotional states. Vegetables and starchy, fibrous foods such as grains, potatoes, beans, corn, and rice are a wonderful source of complex carbohydrates. Tryptophan also increases serotonin production. If you want a good dose of tryptophan, have a slice of turkey or a filet of salmon. Turkey and salmon are also great sources of low-fat protein.

While we're discussing complex carbohydrates and your diet, I want to say a word about wheat. People who are allergic to wheat often report feeling depressed after eating this grain. It has been linked to depression, so you might want to be tested for a wheat allergy. I'm very allergic to wheat and will dive headfirst into a depressed mood if I ingest it. Replace wheat products with spelt, rice, oat or rye breads, crackers, and cereals. Spelt has a wonderful flavor and is very nutritious.

—**Avoid diet sodas and the artificial sweetener aspartame.** Phenylalanine is a major component of the artificial sweetener aspartame, and depressed individuals are often allergic to this amino acid. I have a very dear friend who is extremely allergic to phenylalanine. She recently discovered that her dark moods tended to pop up after consuming any product containing it. For years, she habitually guzzled down one can of diet soda after another.

This particular soda pop contained tons of the artificial sweetener aspartame. No wonder she always felt "blue." Found in most diet sodas, aspartame is also used to sweeten many diet candies, yogurts, cookies, ice creams, and numerous other low-calorie processed foods.

In addition, combination free-form amino acid supplements often contain the amino acid phenylalanine. If you're depressed, check all of your foods and supplements for aspartame or phenylananine.

— **A blue mood or the sugar blues: Is there a relationship?** Pure sugars such as table sugar, corn syrups, and processed brown sugars can add to a gloomy mood. Pure sugars flood our cells and provide us with an immediate burst of energy. This is why we often feel very energized after drinking a sugary soda or eating a candy bar. Sadly, this spurt of energy is short-lived and is usually followed by an intense sensation of fatigue or depression. These sugars exit our bodies as quickly as they invade our cells, leaving us "blue" and exhausted. When this happens, it's not uncommon for us to go after another "hit" of sugar. This starts the cycle all over again, creating an addiction to the mood-altering "high" that sugar provides. Unfortunately, this cycle also traps us into depression. If you're addicted to sugar and are suffering from depression, now is the time to remove this substance from the body. To normalize your blood-sugar levels, take a daily supplement of pure **spirulina algae,** as directed on the label. Spirulina is full of essential vitamins and minerals. Taking 400–500 mcg of **chromium** per day will not only reduce your craving for sugar, but it will help your body metabolize fats for energy.

— **Other supplements to consider for depression.** Begin by correcting any vitamin or mineral deficiencies you have with a good multivitamin. Many depressed people suffer from vitamin and mineral shortages. Let's look at some of the other nutrients that depressed individuals tend to be lacking in.

- **Zinc**—Interestingly, zinc promotes mental alertness. Increase your intake of zinc to 50 mg per day, but make sure that your total intake (from other supplements) does not exceed 100 mg.

- **Vitamin B Complex**—The Bs are essential for proper function of the nervous system and brain. Let's examine the important role that some B vitamins play in combating depression. **Inositol,** also found in the B-complex vitamins, is an important nutrient for serotonin activity. **Folic acid** (found in B-complex) is often deficient in depressed individuals, as is **Vitamin B6.** Take B-complex as directed on the label. For severe depression, ask your doctor about Vitamin B injections. Injections of **Vitamin B12** should also be considered for severe depression. This nutrient fights fatigue by increasing energy levels, and it will also help alleviate a depressed state of mind

- Essential fatty acids—found in **evening primrose, black currant seed oil,** and **flaxseed oil** are necessary for normal brain function and for the transmission of nerve impulses. Take this supplement as directed on the label, and use it in conjunction with 500 IU of **Vitamin E.**

- **Vitamin C** levels should always be increased when one is suffering from depression. Vitamin C is needed to support the immune system and to fend off illness. Stress eats up Vitamin C, and depression is very stressful for the body. Take 500 mg of Vitamin C three times per day. If physical illness sets in, you can increase this dose to 1,000 mg three times per day. Make sure your Vitamin C is buffered.

- **Calcium** is extremely necessary for proper transmission of nerve impulses, and **magnesium** is required for brain function. Both of these minerals have a soothing effect on the nervous system. Take 2,000 mg of calcium with 1,000 mg of magnesium in a chelate form an hour before bed for a restful night's sleep.

Proper nutrition supports the body. When the body is under less stress, this minimizes emotional stress. The herbal world can also assist us in decreasing emotional stress.

(**Note:** Do not use any of the following herbs if you're currently taking an antidepressant. Do not discontinue your antidepressant without the assistance of your health-care provider.)

— For minor depression, try **Gingko biloba.** This particular plant has a long history of use in China, and it's a top-selling remedy in France and Germany. Gingko improves blood circulation to the brain and the central nervous system. This, in turn, helps memory and concentration. For mild depression, take as directed in capsule form.

— For mild to moderate depression, read up on the herb **damiana.** The leaves of this fragrant shrub produce a very pleasant-tasting tea. Because capsules containing damiana are usually comprised of other herbs, use this remedy in a tincture form. Place 25–30 drops in a glass of water or juice 3–4 times per day, or as directed on the label.

— For moderate depression, the plant world has another solution, **St. John's wort.** The petals of these pretty yellow flowers have oil glands that contain hypericin. This constituent turns the oil red. The red-colored hypericin has antidepressant qualities, and it's extremely useful for moderate depression. Herbal research for depression recommends 300 mg of St. John's wort (0.3 percent hypericin) 3 times per day. Improvement in mood will occur in several weeks.

(**Note:** Hypersensitivity to sunlight has been reported by some users of St. John's wort.)

Before we go on, let's explore one more natural remedy for depression. **SAM** or **SAM-e (S-adenosylmethione)** is a nutritional supplement that can work wonders with severe depression. SAM-e appears to increase levels of necessary neurotransmitters such as serotonin, often low in those suffering from depression. SAM-e is not an herb, but an amino acid derivative, found in every single cell in the human body. This nutritional supplement has been used for two decades in 14 countries by doctors treating depression, and has finally made it to the United States. Research on SAM-e continues, and its use in treating severe depression looks promising. Look for this product at your local drug store or health food store.

Recommended doses vary from practitioner to practitioner. As a result, I strongly suggest that you use SAM-e as stated on the label. If you continue to have questions about this nutritional supplement, speak with your health-care practitioner, or consult with a pharmacist.

(**Note:** If you're on medication for severe depression, do not discontinue your medication and switch to SAM-e without first consulting your health-care provider.)

Every year, approximately 11 million of us will be affected by depression. Understanding what contributes to our depressed moods enables us to take action to remedy this emotional state. If you find that after trying the above holistic approach, you're still engulfed in a severe depression, please don't hesitate to reach out for help. You can contact your local United Way Agency or Family Service Center for assistance.

Marianne decided to treat herself to a hot bubble bath. After drawing the water, she added several drops of the essential oils **lavender** and **rose** to the water. Her girlfriend had told her that these scents were useful for relieving depression, and at this point, she was willing to try anything. Marianne lit several rose-scented candles and then gently lowered her body into the comfort of the bath. *Why don't I do things like this for myself more often?* she thought.

As the warm water relaxed her muscles, her mood softened. Laying her head back on the edge of the tub, she closed her eyes and visualized herself before the depression had settled in. As she did so, the tears made their way down her cheeks. "I can't do this by myself," she admitted. "I need some help." Marianne cupped her hands and brought the scented water to her face. After washing her tears away, she suddenly remembered a conversation she'd had with a friend several weeks ago.

Marianne reflected back on her lunch date with Adam. He had just come through a serious depression and had shared with her how he had come out the other side. As she lathered rich oatmeal soap onto her arms, she reflected on what her friend had said: "A holistic health-care provider gave me a hand," he had remarked. Adam's face had beamed as he recounted the path he had taken to make it through this dark time. As he shared his experience, he seemed so serene and at peace with himself. Marianne remembered feeling a bit jealous of him. She had also noticed that he was no longer drinking his favorite diet soda, but taking herbal tea instead.

During their lunch, Adam made a comment, which at the time seemed especially strange. With a smile, he had announced, "You know, today I'm grateful for my depression. I learned a lot about myself and was able to clean up my mental frame of mind, my lifestyle, and my nutritional state. Today, I feel great."

While rinsing the soap off, Marianne said with determination, "I need to call Adam and find out how he crawled out of his emotional dark hole. Maybe his experience will help me."

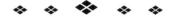

C*hapter three*

RAGING WITH ANGER

It was July, and the heat was stifling. After turning up the air-conditioning, I looked at the middle-aged man sitting on my peach-colored couch. He appeared to be very uncomfortable.

"Is this the first time you've ever visited a therapist?" I asked.

"No," George replied. "When I was married to my ex-wife, Margie, she took me to some quack. You aren't going to tell me I need drugs, are you?"

Surprised, I replied, "Why would you think that?"

Shaking his head in dismay, he said, "The last shrink referred me to another doctor for Prozac, and the stuff made me feel numb, numb as a rock." For a moment, George appeared to be reflecting on his past. "Yep, the therapist thought I was the 'beast,' and that my ex was a poor victim."

Running his fingers through his sandy blond hair, George hesitated and then added, "I have a problem with anger. I just can't seem to control it. This is partially why Margie and I broke up. Now, I have this delightful new woman in my life . . . and last week my anger popped up again. I know I scared her. I don't want to blow this relationship."

"George, what happens when you get angry?" I asked.

Looking a bit ashamed, George replied, "Sometimes I get so mad I punch holes in the wall." Glancing up at me, I could tell he was waiting for a reaction. But he wasn't going to get one from me.

"So, you punch holes in the wall. What else happens?" I questioned.

Casting his eyes downward, he continued, "I just lose it. Totally lose it. I've even screamed at my kids. I know they're frightened of me and I hate that. Now you know why I'm here."

"George," I asked, "are you prepared to do a lot of work?" He appeared confused until I added, "You have a serious rage problem, and, no, drugs will not fix it. Sadly, you've crossed the line from anger to rage, and I bet you've been in this place for some time."

Almost relieved, George replied, "Yes. Now what can I do about it?"

Is George unusual? Absolutely not. In our feeling-denying society, George's plight is very common. Many men and women periodically erupt into a rage. After exploding at spouses, children, lovers, employees, friends, and others, such individuals are then racked with shame about their conduct. Let's begin this chapter by examining the psychology behind raging behavior.

The Psychology of Anger

— **"All I feel is anger."** This is a common sentiment that I hear from clients who have difficulty with rage. Rage attacks appear to come in cycles. A good analogy to a rage attack would be a full teakettle placed on the stove, the water inside of it slowly churning to a boil. After a while, the expanding steam in the kettle must escape. Eventually the steam violently shoots through the nozzle of the kettle, causing it to whistle. If one is not careful, the steam can create a nasty burn.

Rage attacks work just like a steaming teakettle. Over a period of time, little frustrations, irritations, and anger naturally build. For most of us, anger is a normal consequence of living. Sadly, in our society, we're constantly rewarded for not expressing this emotion. Religious institutions, mental healthcare providers, physicians, and contemporary spiritual teachers are quick to tell us that anger is "unhealthy" or "sinful." Anger is only unhealthy if we don't process it appropriately. Not understanding this, many of us don't express our irritations, frustration, and anger as these emotions occur. Instead, we stuff our feelings. Eventually all of this stuffed anger comes to a violent boil.

If we continue to repress our anger, we eventually find ourselves on anger-overload. When we reach this point, anything can, and will, set us off. Explosive rage is a direct consequence of overloaded anger. In order to begin healing from rage attacks, it's extremely important to identify everyday moments of anger.

— **Identifying anger.** For a month, document your daily mood changes. "Impossible!" you say? It may feel that way, but here are a few guidelines to follow. When you feel resentment, frustration, irritation, annoyance, agitation, disgust, or exasperation, guess what? You're angry. For a month, record your daily reactions to stress and upset in an "anger journal." List what brought on these feelings. Who placed added stress on you at home or on the job? Did someone cut in front of you while you were driving to work, or did a family member do something that hurt you? Was a store clerk rude to you? Were your opinions ignored or discounted? Be honest.

— **Look at your body.** Many ragers have difficulty identifying the above emotions. If this is true for you, begin documenting changes in your body. One man I worked with had to get up and urinate every time we talked about his sexual abuse. He was raging but didn't know how to express it. Another raging client broke out in boils when he was mad. One woman had attacks of diarrhea whenever we talked about her ex-husband. My husband also had difficulty with this emotion. When he couldn't express anger, his body would react with an outbreak of acne. Acne breakouts became his "red flag" alert for the anger emotion. Other physical responses to anger include migraine headaches, hemorrhoids, a sudden increase in blood pressure, a rupture of rashes, herpes simplex, nail biting, scab picking, hair pulling, or breaking out in a sweat.

For a month, document bodily changes daily. Also, write about any upsets or disappointments you experienced that day. After a month, go through your calendar to see how your body expresses the emotion of anger. Alcoholism, drug dependence, compulsive eating, anorexia, bulimia, or other addictive behaviors have some of their roots in the emotion of anger. Be sure to list any substances you use in excess, and note when your use increases.

— **Look at your past.** My mother was incapable of expressing anger in a healthy manner. Interestingly, family friends and relatives continue to wonder why she died of cancer at the age of 38. My mother was, essentially, eaten up with stuffed rage.

My father came from a family where there was a lot of unexpressed anger. Silent raging is built-up anger that is never expressed. My grandfather was a very angry man who would repress his rage. Because he never dealt with this anger, my father acted it out—rather loudly, I might add. As you can imagine, I didn't have a clue about venting anger in a healthy fashion.

I either stuffed it like my mother and suffered bouts of colitis, or exploded like dear old Dad, breaking dishes.

Children learn about expressing the emotion of anger by watching their parents and caregivers. On a sheet of paper, describe how your mother handled her anger. Next, look at how your father processed his fury. Finally, describe what your anger looks like. Then, compare your expression of this emotion with that of your parents or other childhood caregivers and relatives. Who are you most like when expressing anger?

— **Old baggage.** Rage attacks can be the result of "over-feelings." George raged at his girlfriend. I wonder how much of his raging had to do with his unfinished business about his ex-wife's history of extramarital affairs. If we haven't totally resolved childhood losses, disappointments, divorces, old job conflicts, deaths, or feelings of past victimization, we are at risk for displacing these emotions on current-day loved ones.

Feelings in the here-and-now can trigger unresolved emotions from the past. Get a sheet of paper and list the rage attacks you've experienced over the last two years. List the people, situations, and places you were raging at. Once you've done so, ask yourself: (1) Did this particular situation or person deserve all of your rage? (2) Does this situation or person remind you of an event from your past? and (3) Was your expression of rage more than was necessary for the situation you initially felt anger about?

Really looking at our behavior begins to provide us with clues as to why we react in the extreme with anger.

— **Get extra help if you need to.** If you find that you're having difficulty exploring your rage by yourself, seek out the assistance of a therapist who isn't afraid of anger. Be sure to shop around. Too many therapists, counselors, psychologists, spiritual counselors, and psychiatrists shame their clients into believing that anger is an unacceptable emotion. Not understanding rage is a result of long-standing repressed anger. These helping professionals often compound the situation by referring raging individuals for medication.

Support groups such as Co-dependency Anonymous (CODAD) or Emotions Anonymous can also provide you with guidance and they're free of charge. In learning how to process rage attacks in a nondestructive, growth-producing manner, lifestyle changes can greatly help. Here are some tips for managing rageful outbursts.

Lifestyle Remedies for Anger

— **A plan for identifying budding rage.** Having a written plan of action that addresses rage can prevent destructive behavior from occurring. When rage begins, the rapid physical rise in the chemical adrenaline often escalates this emotion. Eventually, a raging person is powerless to turn off the destructive outburst. A rage plan assists you in nipping this behavior in the bud before it intensifies. Begin your plan by identifying what your rage looks like as it builds. Do you get headaches, clench your teeth, slam doors, or start to curse? Does your heart pound, or do you begin making a fist? Can you feel the adrenaline rushing through your veins, or does your foot become lead on the gas pedal while driving your car? List all of the emotional and physical changes that occur for you just before you explode into a rage. These characteristics will serve as your warning, or "red flag"system, when you're on the verge of a rage attack.

— **Create a plan of action for handling rage.** This plan should include:
- taking a time-out and leaving the house or office to walk around the block;

- going to a safe place and beating on, or screaming into, pillows; or

- doing something physical such as hitting a punching bag, pounding nails into a board, stomping on soda cans, tearing up phone books, throwing clay balls at the refrigerator, or writing angry letters to those you're upset with.

— **Give loved ones permission to take a time-out.** Share your rage plan with your loved ones or those who live with you. Tell them to leave the scene if they feel you're about to erupt into a rage. If they're in your space while you're raging, they'll be victimized by your outburst. Even if you're angry with them, no one should have to endure the terror of a rage. When raging occurs, spouses need to be instructed to take any children out of the house. Growing up with a raging parent produces children who rage, self-destruct, suffer from hyperactivity, or are depressed. Let your family know that once your raging reaches a certain point, you're powerless to stop it, and that it's in their best interest to leave you alone.

— **Take care of your basic needs.** People who rage are more at risk for doing so if they're not taking care of their basic needs. There's a saying that goes something like this: "Never get too hungry, angry, lonely, or tired." As we've discussed, letting life's frustrations build is a setup for a rage attack. When we don't take time to relax; don't take care of ourselves emotionally, physically, or spiritually; don't get enough sleep; or neglect developing our creative side, we will feel tired and frustrated with life. Life stops feeling joyful; it becomes taxing on our being. This constant sense of frustration eventually leads us to the door of rage.

Nutrition definitely contributes to raging behavior. If we're hungry and our blood sugar has dropped, we'll be more irritable.

Let's look at nutritional factors that can contribute to a raging state of mind.

Nutrition and Herbs for Alleviating Rage Attacks

— **Cut down on the stimulants.** Whenever I'm working with someone who rages, the first nutritional question I ask is, "How much **caffeine** are you taking in?" Caffeine is a known stimulant. Too much caffeine can make us very irritable and edgy. For years my husband was addicted to a particular type of soda pop, loaded with caffeine. The high sugar content in the soda quickly made its way into his cells, giving him a burst of nervous energy. This, combined with the caffeine, made him agitated, irritable, and snappish, unbearable to be around. In addition, the sugar in his "one soda every hour" routine left him uninterested in breakfast or lunch. If you choose to quit drinking caffeine, try taking 500 mg of **bromelain,** 1,500 mg of **calcium,** and 1,000 mg of **magnesium** daily, along with 30 mg of **coenzyme Q10** twice a day for several weeks. This can, hopefully, assist you in minimizing withdrawal symptoms. The herb **feverfew** is also useful.

In addition to caffeine, the **nicotine** found in cigarettes is a stimulant. Cut down on the level of nicotine in your cigarettes. Switch to a lighter brand. If you decide to quit smoking, refer to Chapter 12, where this is discussed in depth. Interestingly, a number of ragers I have worked with have had a steady diet of caffeine, nicotine, or both. Intake of these chemicals must be reduced, and, ideally, eliminated altogether.

— **Three meals a day.** Those plagued with raging rarely take time to nutritionally nurture themselves. Living on a menu of fast foods (high in salt or sugar), greasy fatty foods, and white flour not only leaves one nutritionally starving, but interferes with the body's ability to absorb calcium. Calcium is extremely necessary for proper nerve function. A deficiency in this mineral stresses an already-rattled nervous system.

Start your morning with a glass of juice and some fruit. If you're on the run, grab apples, oranges, berries, peaches, or bananas. Take time to sit down to eat a proper lunch and dinner. Fish with asparagus, turkey with mushrooms and a side of green beans, and barbecued tofu and sugar snap peas are easy meals to put together. Skip the high-fat fries, and go for a baked potato with grilled vegetables. Add a salad to this, one rich in green leafy lettuces. For you meat lovers, lightly stir-fried vegetables with a bit of lean beef or chicken can be most satisfying.

If our bodies are stressed, we will be at risk for raging. Taking the time to prepare a meal can have a calming effect on the mind. You don't have to be the "Galloping Gourmet" to put together a decent menu. The market is flooded with cookbooks providing recipes for quick, nutritious breakfasts, lunches, and dinners. Go to the bargain table of any major bookstore and pick up a copy of a cookbook that looks interesting to you.

Finally, take time to chew your food. Slow down long enough to appreciate the many flavors and textures of the foods you ingest. Prayer or a silent meditation before eating helps us to appreciate the bounty of foods our planet provides for us.

— **Carrot juice.** Juice carrots with either a pear, apple, a handful of grapes, or strawberries. Today's juicers are very easy to use and can be found in most department stores. Because carrot juice can regulate blood-sugar levels, it guards against hypoglycemia, which often leads to mood swings and rage. I find that popping into the local health food store or vegetarian restaurant for a glass of carrot juice can keep my emotions on an even keel.

— **Supplements, please.** Many ragers go, go, go, and live very stressed lifestyles. This stress depletes the body of essential vitamins and minerals. Rage attacks cause further nutritional depletion. All this does is promote more raging behavior.

Learning how to set time aside to prepare meals is extremely important, but this will take time. In the meantime, make sure you're taking a good, solid multivitamin on a daily basis. Be sure it contains the antioxidant **selenium.**

Stress and rage burn up **Vitamin C,** leaving the immune system vulnerable to colds and other illnesses. To maintain good health, supplement your diet with 2,000–4,000 mg of Vitamin C per day. To prevent stomach irritation, make sure your Vitamin C is buffered, and take it in three separate doses.

Don't forget the significance of **B vitamins**. Every single one of the "Bs" is necessary for the proper function of the nervous system. Take one B-complex vitamin per day.

Heart and blood-pressure difficulties also can plague ragers. A daily dose of 500 IUs of **Vitamin E** will not only help you lower your blood pressure, but will aid in preventing cardiovascular disease and cancer. Each of these illnesses have been tied to both stress factors and to unresolved anger. Deficiencies in this nutrient have also been linked to breast and bowel cancer.

(**Note:** If you have high blood pressure, start by taking a daily dose of 200 IUs of Vitamin E. Slowly increase your dose over a period of three months. Also, if you're taking an anticoagulant medication, check with your health-care provider before using this supplement.)

When rage is a problem, a little extra pantothenic acid or **Vitamin B6** can be of great assistance. Taking 500 mg of this particular anti-stress vitamin can help the overworked thymus gland. It's also good for your nerves and your hair. Speaking of nerves, most ragers seem to be emotionally living on the edge, 24 hours a day. Instead of turning to alcohol, tranquilizers, or other pharmaceutical mood-altering drugs, there are several herbs that can normalize and support the nervous system.

— Let's calm the mind. Skullcap was once called "mad dog" and was thought to cure rabies. Although some of us may look like a mad dog when we're raging, we don't have to have rabies in order to benefit from this herb. Skullcap supports the nervous system, but it doesn't have serious sedative effects. Take in capsule form as directed on the label.

Damiana, known as a Mayan aphrodisiac, can also assist in regulating the nervous system. Use in a glycerin tincture form, and take as directed on the label.

I rarely suggest using **valerian root** because it's a powerful herb and can have toxic effects if it's misused. Because rage attacks can be violent and intense, I'm going to include this remedy in this particular herbal list. If valerian root is not used as directed, it can create serious difficulties. When using this herb for rage attacks, be sure to stick to the suggested dosages. Valerian is most effective when taken before an attack, when the "red flag" signal rage is surfacing. Use in a glycerin tincture form as directed. Put the drops under the tongue for quick absorption. Then, take a time-out. Get away from everyone, and find a quiet space. As the valerian root tincture makes its way into your bloodstream, try to meditate on scenery that brings you peace of mind, such as an oceanfront, the mountains, or a favorite bubbling brook of fresh water.

(**Note:** Do not use any of these herbs if you're taking traditional sleep medications, tranquilizers, or antidepressants.)

— Those headaches. Headaches often come before or immediately after a rage attack. In England, a stick of **marshmallow** was given to teething toddlers to suck on. Plato knew about this herb, and now you, too, can enjoy its many benefits. Marsh mallow is used anytime the mucous membranes need to be soothed. Used in combination with **feverfew,** it's an ideal remedy for headaches. Feverfew has long been utilized by herbalists as a treatment for migraine headaches. Visit your local health food store for tablets containing both the herbs feverfew and marshmallow. Be sure you use this remedy as directed on the label.

— **Breathe and release.** Breathing in, and then releasing, can have a calming effect on your physical and emotional well-being, especially before a rage attack hits. Essential oils can also assist in calming down a brewing rage. For years, I've had the essential herbal oils **lavender, rosemary**, and **frankincense** on hand at all times. I have vials of the oils in the kitchen, bedroom, bathroom, office, and in my purse for those sudden rageful flare-ups. When the intense emotion of rage begins to surface, take a tissue and put several drops of these essential oils on it. Take a time-out and breathe in the scents. Purple lavender has a wonderful reputation for relieving both headaches and irritability. Rosemary is one of my favorite scents. This fragrance is uplifting, and its fresh outdoors smell quickly clears a foggy mind. Frankincense was used 5,000 years ago to honor the Egyptian sun god, Ra. This luxuriously scented herb has been used in religious rituals for thousands of years.

Here is a visualization to use when breathing in essential oils:

Imagine that your rage is bright red. Give the scent of your essential oil the color blue. With each inhalation, imagine the blue color of the fragrance from the herb slowly entering into your body. As you exhale, visualize this healing color pushing out the red rage within you.

Keep doing this visualization until you've calmed down. This is one of my favorite quick-fix meditations, and I continue to use it to this day.

Too many people in our society today try to ignore their anger. Is it any wonder that road rage, gun violence, and domestic abuse continue to make the headlines of our newspapers? Anger is a normal, natural human emotion, but it continues to be viewed by many as a sign of weakness, a lack in spiritual evolution, and a sin. Pushing this feeling away will not make it disappear. Like the steam in the teakettle, pent-up rage will eventually makes its escape and "burn" you. Learning how to properly process anger takes time and courage. Old, negative messages about this strong emotion must be rewritten and redefined. Using a holistic approach to address the problem of rage can make the path of healing easier and enlightening. If you'd like to learn more about the healthy expression of anger, pick up a copy of the book *The Dance of Anger* by Harriet G. Lerner.

As we left my office and began the trek down the stairs to the waiting room, George asked, "Am I hopeless?"

Smiling at him, I said, "Heavens, no. You didn't put a hole in my wall when I confronted you, did you?"

Surprised, George asked, "Someone actually put a hole in your wall?"

"Yep," I replied. "Someone put a huge hole in my wall. Thankfully, she's learned how to handle her anger as it comes up and hasn't put a hole in a wall for quite some time."

With this, George's eyes got very big. "She?" he asked. "I thought only men did stuff like that."

Chuckling, I answered, "Of course, 'she.' Women can get just as mad as men. You do have a lot to learn about anger." Both of us began to laugh.

As I opened the door leading out to the front yard, George shook my hand and said, "Yes, I do have much to learn. Guess I'll see you next week. It's good to know that there are others like me, and that a few of them have been able to heal. This gives me hope."

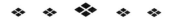

PART II

Healing Through Relationships

❦ ❦ ❦ ❦

*C*hapter *four*

LOVE DEPENDENCY VERSUS
HEALTHY SELF-LOVE

"**D**enise, what on earth are you talking about?" Lea was on the phone with her younger sister. Denise was extremely distressed, but Lea didn't know why.

"I just can't believe you left that message on my recorder," Denise wailed.

Oh, heavens, thought Lea. *What is she talking about?*

"How could you say something like that when you knew he would be listening?" Denise sobbed.

Now Lea was very confused, and so she asked, "What message on what recorder? I leave tons of phone messages for you." She then added, "Honey, you're going to have to be more specific about why you're so upset."

There was a minute of silence, and then Denise answered, "You left a message on my recorder saying you didn't think Al was being very understanding. He heard it and became furious. How could you be so insensitive? He isn't that bad. Now he's mad at me. How could you?" With this, she began to cry again.

Lea shook her head and sighed. She had thought Denise's private phone line was still tied in to her personal message service. Lea had no idea that her sister's boyfriend had access to these messages. After gathering her wits, she replied, "First of all, I wasn't aware that you were now sharing a message recorder with Al. Second, when you told me he wasn't talking to you and had hurt your feelings, I became very alarmed."

"I said that?" asked Denise.

Lea was surprised that her sister had forgotten this phone conversation. "Yes," she added, "and there's more. Later that day, you called me a second time. Once again I heard how distressed you were over your relationship with Al. Then you said, 'He was so inconsiderate, but if I tell him how I really feel, he'll threaten to leave.' This led me to believe that all is not well. What did you expect? I get concerned about you. Are you standing up for yourself?"

To this, her sister replied, "Well, no. My problem is that I'm afraid to be honest. If I do say what I need to say, I'm terrified he'll walk out on me. Then I'll be all alone, and I just can't live without him."

Love-dependent individuals have great difficulty getting their needs met in their relationships and are upset because they believe that their "significant other" should recognize this. It's as if the love-dependent person and the partner are living on two separate planets. At this point, you might be asking, "Why is this?" The psychology behind love dependence can provide many clues.

The Psychology of Love-Dependent Relationships

— **Overdoers.** Love-dependent individuals look outside themselves for love, hoping this will fill up their painful sense of emptiness. Sadly, this rarely works. The insatiable need for love is the result of our inability to love ourselves. This lack of self-love perpetuates dependent love in relationships.

By overdoing, working just a little harder at pleasing others and giving more of ourselves, we assume we'll be loved. We also believe that if we just do and give enough, we won't be abandoned by our significant others. Unfortunately, instead of creating mutually respecting partnerships, we end up feeling even more empty and needy.

In my private practice as a Licensed Marriage and Family Therapist, I work with a number of men and women who are in very sad relationships. These folks are usually extremely loving human beings who tend to "give till it hurts." In some cases, they will put the wants and desires of others before their own basic needs.

Every relationship has periodic problems. This is a normal part of the human condition. If these difficulties are resolved as they come up, this protects the relationship from dysfunction. Love-dependent individuals fear honest communication and tend to push normal intimacy difficulties underground, in the hope that this will fix relationship problems.

Not only is there difficulty in standing up for ourselves with a significant other, but problems also exist with children, friends, relatives, community activities, and religious organizations. Saying no feels impossible, and the fear of conflict forces us to constantly give in to the wants of others. The thought is, *I don't want to be unloved by anyone.*

Why can't we say no? Many of us believe we don't have a right to say no to others. In essence, we don't recognize that we deserve to be treated as we treat others. On an unconscious level, we don't seem to understand that we're entitled to the same nurturing that we give to our partners, children, and friends. Why is this? Let's look and see.

Take out a piece of paper and list the many different things you've done for your partner, children, family, extended family, friends, co-workers, pets, religious organization, and community over the past month. After you've made this list, go back and document how much time was spent doing each of these tasks. Next, make a list of the things you've done for yourself this month. How much time did you spend on *you?* Do you spend enough time taking care of yourself? If not, write out how you can change this situation. (Here's a hint on how to complete this task: Are you doing for yourself what you're doing for others?)

Primary relationships and the fear of abandonment. For some of us, the thought of living alone is frightening. "What would I do without her?" "I need to know he's there," "I can't start all over again," or "I'll just die if she leaves me" are the statements of distress I hear from people who are absolutely terrified of being alone. For some, the mere thought of not being with a particular person can create a sense of panic. The belief is, "Without her, I'm nothing. She makes my life complete," or "What will I have to live for if he's gone?"

Love-dependent people feel that they "need" a relationship, just like they need to eat and breathe. In a functional relationship, partners don't feel that they desperately need each other. Instead, they *choose* to be together. In a healthy relationship, desperate need, dishonesty, lack of communication, and a sense of power-lessness are replaced with a respect for individual likes and dislikes, worthy goals, honesty, an agreement to periodically disagree, tolerance, and a commitment to self-growth.

Are love-dependent people weak-willed and lacking in character? No, this is a misconception. They often tend to be very high-functioning creative thinkers who are capable of accomplishing several tasks at once. Unfortunately, they're unable to appreciate the beautiful essence of themselves and find it necessary to be in a relationship in order to feel whole.

Take out a piece of paper and write the word *ALONE* in big letters at the top of the page. Next, write down what comes to mind when you think of this word. Are you frightened? Do you feel uneasy? Do you begin to feel a sense of panic?

Now, write an essay about living without your partner.

As you write it, let yourself cry if you need to. After you're done, find a friend or therapist to share your story with. Then brainstorm with this person about what you would do if you found yourself living without this partner. List those actions you would need to take financially, emotionally, environmentally (moving to a new home), and legally (in case of divorce, separation, or death). If you have children, be sure to address what you would need to do to take care of their needs. After completing this task, you will realize that you're more capable of surviving on your own than you think. Understanding this concept, it's now time to learn how to set boundaries with your partner.

Learning to say no. Love-dependent individuals tend to have no time for themselves because they can't say no to the demands of others. Because the fear of saying no is often very strong, it's difficult to set limits with others. "If I tell him not to talk to me that way, he won't speak to me at all," or "I'll pay the price if I ask her to cut down on her spending" are statements that are also saying, "I don't want to rock the boat and upset this person because she or he might retaliate by abandoning me." Are these fears real? Sometimes yes, but often no.

My husband, Michael, and I work with couples as a team. We've found that, typically, one member of the couple is usually oblivious to any hurt feelings or serious difficulties in the relationship. In therapy, we often ask couples to make a list of all of the complaints they have about each other. When these are read out loud, one or both individuals are often surprised by what they hear. Responses can range from, "I didn't know that hurt you. You never told me you felt that way," to "Why didn't you let me know this was a problem? I never had any idea you were so upset." Why are such complaints a surprise? As mentioned earlier, in dependent relationships, one or both partners will tiptoe around their mate or never set boundaries or express their true feelings.

A good exercise is to make a list of all of the things you would like to express to your partner but have never had the courage to say. For example, "I'm hurt that you don't help me around the house," or "I feel angry when you make fun of my weight," or "I feel lonely when you don't listen to me." After you've done so, put the complaints into letter form. Now close your eyes, visualize your partner, and imagine telling this person that you have some things to share. Let your partner know that although you must share your feelings with them, they don't necessarily have to agree with you. Before opening your eyes and sharing your written words, imagine yourself saying, "Please don't interrupt me while I'm reading this." As you read your letter out loud, cry if you need to. This is very normal. After you've completed this task, read your letter to a friend, therapist, or spiritual advisor. Be sure to share this note with someone who will be supportive of you.

When you're feeling especially brave, leave this letter for your partner to read. Do this at a time when your mate will be alone so you don't have to be present for their initial reaction to your letter. After your partner has had time to read your note, telephone your partner and ask, "How did you feel about it?" Telephoning gives you some distance. In this way, you can feel out any intense reaction to your letter before meeting face-to-face. After talking on the phone, meet in person in a public place to discuss your letter. A quiet restaurant or park works well. See if the two of you can resolve some of these issues. If this doesn't work, you may need mediation from a third party, such as a marriage therapist, spiritual advisor, or mentoring couple.

Love dependence is fostered by dishonesty, while honest communication with self and others enhances self-love. "Getting honest" about a primary relationship can be difficult. The thought of openly discussing unresolved issues can set off the "what ifs." The fear of what will happen if honest sharing takes place often keeps us from saying what we need to say to those we love. In most cases, the "what ifs" never materialize. Instead, the honest sharing creates an opportunity for healing, both within the relationship and on an individual basis. When complaints are openly aired, boundaries can be established, and healthy intimacy can begin to replace dependence.

Self-love—the basis for a healthy relationship. To have a healthy, loving relationship, we must first know how to love ourselves. In my family system, it's important for me to take care of my needs before those of the relationship. If I don't do so, I can't be a healthy participant in a relationship. Instead, I will probably expect my partner to fill me up. This is an extreme expectation. Before we can enjoy our relationship as a couple, Michael and I must individually do whatever is necessary to maintain healthy self-love.

After self-love comes the health of the relationship. Michael and I are both responsible for maintaining the well-being of our union. We must often consciously take time away from children, family, and our business to accomplish this goal. A healthy, intimate connection needs continual attention. If we don't take care of our relationship needs, air complaints, and periodically reexamine the boundaries in our partnership, we can't be healthy parents for our children. When we're not taking care of the marriage, we're both at risk for trying to get our emotional needs met through our kids. This isn't fair to the children. Kids need parents, and it's difficult to be a parent if we're trying to be a "best friend."

After looking at the above, it's easy to see that the basis of all healthy relationships depends on whether or not we're able to love ourselves. Let's look at those lifestyle changes that can facilitate this aim.

Lifestyle Remedies for Love-Dependent Individuals

— **Learning how to nurture yourself.** Those of us who are dependent on relationships for our own sense of self-worth often smother those we love. Also, our overdoing can drive our loved ones nuts. Believing that all our self-worth should come from taking care of our partner, our children, or others is very unhealthy. As a result, it's important for us to increase our involvement in self-nurturing activities.

One woman I know convinced herself she had given up sculpting for her husband, children, and community. She said, "I'm so busy taking care of others that I have absolutely no time for sculpting." You might be saying to yourself, "Well, she *should* devote her time to her family." However, sculpting was her passion, and she loved putting her hands in clay. By not taking sculpting time for herself, she was unable to "recharge" her batteries. As a result of not nurturing herself, she wasn't able to be there for her family in a healthy way.

Giving yourself time to dabble in hobbies is very healing. My family knows that I must write at least an hour a day. If I don't take care of this creative need, I feel as if I haven't taken care of *me*. This spills over into my feelings about taking care of *them*.

Attending support groups such as Love Addicts Anonymous or Co-dependents Anonymous can teach us how to begin meeting our own emotional needs. Yes, we do deserve some of the time we're giving to others. One hour once or twice a week at a support group is a good beginning.

Taking care of the basics. My grandmother rarely sat down to eat with us. During mealtimes, she was up and about, serving everyone. All of us were capable of tending to ourselves, but my grandmother felt she needed to take care of *us*. Rarely did I see her eat a full meal herself. Instead, she would pick at the leftovers as she washed the dishes.

Do you take care of *your* basic needs? To determine whether you are, answer the following questions:

- Are you taking the time to eat nutritious foods?
- When you need medical attention, will you visit a health-care provider, or do you put it off?
- Are you getting the rest you need at night?
- Do you set time aside each day to mellow out and unwind? Will you allow yourself a moment of rest with a cup of tea?
- Are there people in your life you can turn to when you need to talk about your frustrations? Can you receive, as opposed to always giving?
- What about exercise? Do you take time to go for short walks or bicycle rides? Is there an activity, such as sailing, swimming, martial arts, folk dancing, or yoga, that you wish you had time for? If so, what is stopping you from exploring this activity?

If you're not taking care of the basics, you won't be able to replenish yourself. Operating on "empty" leaves us feeling resentful, unappreciated, alone, discounted, and unloved. This also sets us up for physical illnesses. When we're emotionally spent, our immune system is lowered.

On a piece of paper, write down what you're willing to do this week to begin taking care of your basic needs, and then follow through on this task. Part of taking care of the basics is knowing what you require in order to stay nutritionally fit. With this in mind, it's time to look at your diet.

Nutrition and Herbs for Assisting
Love-Dependent Individuals

— **For the love of food.** When it comes to diet, love-dependent individuals usually do one of two things: They either eat too much or too little. In most cases, when they do eat, their selection of edibles consists of overprocessed foods. Why do they choose these foods? Overprocessed, sugary, greasy foods are mood-altering and comforting. It's not uncommon for many of us to reach out for our favorite comfort foods when we feel neglected, abandoned, lonely, alienated, taken for granted, and hurt. Love-dependent individuals do this for a very important reason.

It's well known among nutritionists and food-disorder experts that the ingestion of sugar can change how we feel. Starchy carbohydrates also have a temporary calming effect on the senses. If we're feeling unappreciated or misunderstood, a big chocolate chip cookie always comes to mind.

Most love-dependent persons don't know how to process the anger and pain they're feeling. On an unconscious level, they've learned that these "eat treats" will temporarily remove them from the emotional pain they're experiencing. This is how such foods serve a purpose.

On the flip side, when distressed or down, there are those love-dependent individuals who don't eat. Not eating is also very mood altering. When the body is deprived of necessary nutrients, this changes the chemistry of our physical self. In turn, this greatly impacts our emotional state of mind. We become numb and don't have to feel.

For the next month, make a daily journal of what you eat. At the end of each day, look at your list of foods and ask yourself how each of these items affects your mood. What does coffee do for you? Do you feel better after that mid-morning doughnut or pastry? How about lunch? Will you go for a skimpy iceberg lettuce salad or a hamburger and fries? How do you feel after eating these foods—in control, nurtured, or zoned out? Are you one of those people who doesn't eat all day long, but then binges on a big meal at night? Just what do your eating habits look like?

Next, go back over your daily journal and ask yourself, "When during the day was I feeling unattractive, neglected, old, abandoned, useless, unacceptable, hurt, angry, frustrated, neglected, inadequate, shamed, or frightened?" Try to see if there's a connection between your daily moods and the foods you choose to eat. Many of the love-dependent people I work with report that they're most likely to go after comfort foods or not eat at all when they're at odds with a partner. As one woman said to me, "He forgot my birthday, so I made my own cake and ate half of it."

— Self-love equals healthy foods for the body. Most of us think that we know what a healthy diet consists of. Unfortunately, many of us rarely follow nutritious eating plans. Why? There's an unconscious thinking pattern that many love-dependent people play again and again that can set up self-destructive food behaviors. This thought pattern says to us, *My partner is not there for me. I must be unworthy. If my partner refuses to care for me, why should I bother taking care of myself?*

This negative thought pattern must be replaced with an affirmation that says: *I have a right to exist. I deserve emotional, physical, and spiritual health. I now understand that nobody can make me feel whole and complete. Only I can do this. Today, I will start to love myself by properly feeding my body.*

How should you feed yourself? Those of you reading this chapter will have a number of different eating behaviors. As a result, I'm not going to recommend a specific food plan here. Instead, decide for yourself if you're an overeater or an undereater. If you feel you eat too many overprocessed, sugary, fatty foods, refer to Chapter 14, "Obsessive-Compulsive Eating." Even if you feel that you're not overweight, this chapter will give you some wonderful dietary and herbal suggestions. The food plan is simple and easy to implement. If you tend to undereat, refer to Chapter 15, "Anorexia: A Slow Death." Although you may not be suffering from this particular food disorder, the nutritional recommendations and herbal remedies in this chapter work well for undereaters.

Some of you may be in the throes of menopause or may suffer from severe PMS. These conditions only intensify the emotions associated with love dependence. During menopause and PMS, hormones can wreak havoc on our self-esteem and thinking patterns. Combined with love dependence, such conditions can leave us feeling extremely depressed, hopeless, and helpless. When we support the hormonal fluctuations of menopause and PMS with proper foods and certain medicinal herbs, we find that we're in a better position to work through the emotional stress of a love-dependent relationship. If you're suffering mood swings from hormonal fluctuations, turn to Chapter 17: "Premenstrual Syndrome: An Opportunity to Heal," or to Chapter 18: "Menopause: It Isn't a Mental Illness." Regardless of your eating patterns, understand that most love-dependent people tend to have issues with food. Taking the necessary steps to rectify this problem is a true act of self-love.

Love dependence is detrimental to our mental state, physical being, and spiritual development. If we pin all of our hopes and dreams on one person, we're setting ourselves up for a big fall. When feeling empty inside, we must look to ourselves for healing. We can't expect our lovers, husbands, partners, children, parents, or friends to fill us up. We can look to our partner and adult relationships for support, but we must learn to love and nurture ourselves.

All of us possess a divine spark. This spark of divinity resides deep within us and is at the core of our being. For the love-dependent person, finding this spark is the challenge that lies ahead.

Although Denise had calmed down, she continued talking about her relationship with her boyfriend. Lea bit her tongue as she listened to her sister tell her how unappreciative Al had been. "If only he would change, then I could be happy. Why doesn't he see that? As long as he continues to act this way, I'm going to be miserable," lamented Denise.

Lea took a deep breath and said, "He can't make you happy. Only *you* can do that. Are you going to spend the rest of your life waiting for him to change?"

With this confrontation, there was utter silence on the other end of the phone. After several moments, Denise abruptly responded with, "Are you taking his side?"

"No," replied Lea sadly. "Right now I'm concerned about *you*. When are you going to do what you need to make yourself happy? It's an inside job, and no one can do this for you. No man can make you complete."

Lea then heard a sob escape from her sister. Denise admitted, "Yes, you're right. I've spent years hoping he would 'get it,' and I'm miserable. Nothing has changed for me because I keep waiting for him to make the first move. I guess it's time for me to do something different, but I'm scared."

With this, Lea remembered the path she had fearfully trudged as she began her own healing from love dependence. She confessed, "I was scared, too, but I survived. Now I can be here to support *you* on your journey."

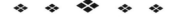

Chapter five

DIVORCE: THE END OF A DREAM

Eric was devastated, and his sister Pauline knew it. As she watched him play with her two-year-old son, Stuart, she poured some lemon balm herbal tea for both of them and thought, *Behind that false front is a man about to fall apart.* Pauline then returned to the kitchen counter to get the tray of egg-salad sandwiches for her brother. "Here. Eat. You look like a rail," she said as she piled his plate high with a couple of sandwiches and a huge spoonful of salad.

"Whoa! That's enough. Are you trying to give me a heart attack? There must be a pound of mayonnaise in that egg salad. Not to mention the gob of cholesterol in the eggs. Do you eat like this all of the time?" he laughed, as he picked at his lunch.

"No," she replied. "I use low-fat canola oil mayonnaise and crumbled tofu, in combination with just a few eggs, so just calm down." Looking at the circles under his eyes, she added, "Eric, you look just awful. Obviously you aren't taking care of yourself at all."

Pauline sat down to mash a bit of banana on her plate. As she began to spoon-feed the fruit to Stuart, she asked her brother, "Have you seen Marilyn lately?" Before she finished her sentence, Pauline regretted opening her mouth. Suddenly, Eric's whole mood changed. The false front fell from his face, and Pauline could tell that her brother was very upset.

Eric put down his sandwich and gazed out the window. He and Marilyn had once had so many goals to look forward to. Sadly, those dreams would never materialize. At that moment, he missed her terribly. *How could she do this to us? To me? To our girls?* he thought angrily. Marilyn had filed for divorce just the week before. This move had totally shocked him. Never in a million years would he have believed that his wife would do this to him. Eric had always told Marilyn that she reminded him of an angel, his angel sent from above. Today, his angel was nowhere to be found, and nothing could fill up the emptiness.

In America, more than two million people a year experience the trauma and loss of divorce. Divorce creates a well of intense emotions for the couple ending a marriage, and the feelings related to such an experience must be processed. If these emotions are ignored, three lifelong consequences will result. First, when a divorced individual doesn't work through unresolved concerns about an ex, chances are that the person will eventually find her- or himself in a similar relationship in the future. Second, if strong emotions and problems in a past marriage are disregarded, this baggage can often surface in a subsequent love affair. Third, if parents don't take responsibility for healing from divorce, any secrets or stuffed emotions from the marriage will be acted out by the children. Unresolved divorce issues can impact everyone caught up in this drama, leaving lifelong scars. In order to recover and not repeat this scenario in the future, it's important to examine the psychology behind divorce.

The Psychology of Divorce

— **The end of the couple.** Anytime we experience the termination of a relationship, we're confronted with a grief issue. Even if there's a feeling of relief, the original dream of what the marriage could have been must be grieved for. To understand this concept more fully, try the following visualization:

> *Find a quiet spot to sit where you won't be disturbed. Close your eyes and take several deep breaths. As you breathe in, imagine that your cleansing breath is blue, and that it permeates every cell of your body. When you exhale, visualize this breath as red stress leaving your body. Slowly breathe in and out for several minutes. Next, in your mind's eye, remember what you looked like on the day of your wedding. How old were you when you said "I do"? Were you excited on this day? Joyous and full of hope? What were your dreams as you stood next to your new mate, reciting vows of love and dedication? Notice how you feel as you focus on your wedding day. Do you cry? Are you hurt? Does your chest tighten up? Are you irritated? Frightened? Excited or angry? How do you feel when you reflect on this younger version of yourself?*

Open your eyes and write about the feelings you had during this meditation. Any intense emotions experienced indicate that you have unfinished business with this marriage. Grief consists of many emotions, but the most prevalent are sadness and anger. If you feel these emotions about current or past-day marital issues, you have unresolved grief that is in need of your attention. Sadness about the loss of the dream your marriage represented on your wedding day is also a major grief issue.

— **Resentment.** Whenever a marriage terminates, it has usually ended because of many unresolved feelings of resentment. Infidelity, addiction, in-laws, money issues, children, abuse, a sense of not being appreciated or feeling taken for granted, and sex issues are just a few of the forms of marital resentment expressed by newly divorced individuals visiting my office. Just because your partner is no longer living with you doesn't mean that your resentment is gone.

Think of all of the things your ex-partner has done that have made you angry. List these issues on a piece of paper. Next, write a letter to your ex about them. You don't have to send this letter, but this task is necessary for your healing. In your letter, tell this person why you're angry, irritated, frustrated, disgusted, or annoyed with them. Curse if you must. Say whatever it is you need to say. If possible, read this letter to a friend or therapist. You can also read it out loud to yourself. Do so while looking at yourself in the mirror, and let your tears flow if you need to. If you find that your anger is overwhelming, beat on pillows, rip up paper, go hit golf balls, or throw Nerf balls at the wall. Discharge this anger from your body. Stuffed anger directly affects your immune system and other bodily functions. To deny that you're angry when you're seething inside is destructive to your being.

Also, when we deny our anger, it can move inward and turn into a dark depression, migraine headaches, colitis, backaches, or a host of other disorders. By doing the above task, you can learn how to express your anger in a productive, healthy manner.

— **Saying good-bye.** Even though the relationship has ended, there will always be a part of you that remembers "the dream." It's extremely important for you to grieve for this dream. Discharging grief from the body is just as important as processing anger. Unexpressed grief also lowers the immune system and can lead to colds; viruses; and chest, head, or nasal congestion. Here is another meditation that will assist you in moving through your grief:

Close your eyes and remember once more what you and your ex-partner looked like when you were newly married. In your mind's eye, spend some time visually scrutinizing the younger version of your ex-mate. During the early years of your relationship, what did you appreciate about this person? Imagine you and your ex-partner alone, together, enjoying each other's company. Watch the two of you interact. Is there love? Compassion?

During this same visualization, ask yourself what it is you regret about this marriage ending. Do you regret that the two of you could not resolve your differences or that this individual wouldn't do anything about a dysfunctional behavior? Possibly you regret that the two of you could not grow old together, raise your family as a couple, or build the business or new home you had planned.

Write a second letter to your ex-partner, telling him or her what you liked about them. In this particular letter, you also need to communicate what you regret about the relationship ending. For example; "I really did appreciate your creativity and regret that I will not get to explore this with you," or "I loved the way you parented our children and am saddened that you will no longer be a consistent presence in their lives." After you've composed this letter, read it to a friend, therapist, or out loud to yourself as you look in the mirror.

When looking at life traumas and their impact on our well-being, divorce is right up there with the death of a loved one. The above steps can provide you with the tools you will need to begin healing emotionally from your divorce. At this time, you may also find it useful to visit a professional mental health-care provider. Such a person can aid you in moving through your emotions, as well as some of the lifestyle changes you will be confronted with. Lifestyle changes always accompany divorce. Different households, child visitation times, financial issues, and awkward social moments can create a great deal of stress for the newly divorced person. Let's look at some lifestyle changes that will aid you in making the transition from "couple" to single person.

Lifestyle Remedies for Divorce

— **Photographs and mementos: Pack them up!** Years ago, I was engaged to be married to my high school sweetheart. At that time, I was desperately in love with him and was looking forward to being his wife. When I found out he was having an affair, I thought that my life was over. Looking at photographs of us together around my house constantly brought tears to my eyes and reduced me to an emotional puddle. Every time I saw a reminder of our time together, this triggered overwhelming emotion, making it difficult to carry on with the tasks of everyday living.

Such personal memorabilia can keep us in a constant state of emotional upset, making healing more difficult. During this tender time, it's important that you not be constantly bombarded with reminders of the relationship. Although you must feel the feelings and process this loss, there is a proper time and place for this. Because you still have day-to-day responsibilities to attend to, the following lifestyle change is suggested: Search your wallet, your house, place of work, and yard for any clothing, photographs of your ex-partner or the two of you, and personal belongings or other keepsakes. Stack them on your kitchen table, then allow yourself a block of quiet time to go through these articles. Remember days gone by, and let yourself experience your feelings for as long as you need to.

After you have done so, take the photographs and make copies of them for later use. When doing anger work, it's often therapeutic to write your ex an angry letter and then burn or tear it up with this set of pictures. Put the copies in a file in your closet or in a drawer. Then place the rest of the items from your relationship (gifts, jewelry, cards, love letters) in a box.

Seal the box with tape, and put this in your attic, garage, or cellar. In one year, you will be in a different space, emotionally and physically. Because you will have healed a bit from the trauma of divorce, you'll be in a better place to determine which of these mementos you want to keep.

If your children are living with you, it's appropriate for you to tell them they can keep out any photographs or items from their other parent in their room. Let them know you're doing what you need to do to heal, but that this should not in any way keep them from continuing to love and appreciate the other parent.

— **Rearrange your bedroom.** For a married couple, the bedroom represents love, sex, quiet talks, and precious moments spent together. If you continue to live in the house you shared with your ex-partner, recognize that your bedroom is now your room— your room alone. It's imperative that you transform this room into a comfortable living space for *you*. With a touch of paint and a little time spent rearranging furniture, you can create a room that is emotionally safe. An inexpensive new comforter or afghan can make all the difference in the world.

— **Distinguish grief time from isolation.** In the 1970s, divorce was looked down upon by society at large. As a result, my poor mother felt a great deal of shame about being divorced. She even said to me, "We don't need to let everyone know about this. Family laundry is family laundry." I was told to keep my parents' divorce to myself because "What would the neighbors think?" Initially, this mentality kept my mother from socializing with her friends. To this day, I remember her isolating herself in her blue-on-blue bedroom.

You'll need alone time to grieve and heal, but try to avoid isolating yourself from loving friends and family. Right now you need the support of those loved ones. Continue to attend the religious institution of your choice, and don't give up your hobbies or withdraw from support groups. Surround yourself with people who will let you be sad or mad when you need to be.

— **Exercise.** After experiencing the emotional drain of a divorce, the idea of exercise can seem impossible. In spite of this, don't put the sweat pants and tennis shoes away. Exercise will give you an emotional break from the feelings that accompany the breakup of a significant relationship. By focusing on activities such as jogging, aerobics, bike-riding, fast-paced walking, weight lifting, dance, swimming, golfing, or whatever grabs your interest, you will be able to take a small vacation, emotionally and physically, from your divorce. Yoga and meditation can also provide you with some much-needed relief from the stress you're experiencing.

— **Get creative.** Expressing our emotions through music, painting, drawing, sculpting, cooking, sewing, writing, mechanical tinkering, poetry, or any other creative venture has been life-saving for many famous people throughout history. Over the centuries, writers have expressed their pain on paper, and the emotions of some of our most brilliant artists can be seen on canvas. Listen to a piece of classical music, and see if you can *feel* the notes of music. Expression of emotions through creativity can be a spiritually healing experience. If you've stopped playing the piano or have let that bag of sculpting clay dry up, get busy. Take out the sheet music, grab the pen or paints, and release your feelings about your divorce, using some form of creativity.

When we end a relationship, not only do we tend to neglect our emotional state and spirit, but also our physical well-being.

In our grief, we stop taking care of ourselves nutritionally. Here are a few simple nutritional rules to follow during this hard time.

Nutrition and Herbs to Assist the Divorced Individual

— **Balancing out the fast-food habit.** How often I have heard from newly divorced people, "I'll just grab a burger or a slice of pizza on my way home." Before the ink is dry on the divorce decree, the nutritional state of both parties has often sunk to an all-time low. "It's only me. Why should I cook?" and "I get the kids fed and just don't feel like putting energy into doing the same for myself" is a common excuse for not eating right. One woman told me that her dinner consisted of popcorn and diet sodas. Because I know you won't initially take the time to create healthy meals for yourself, I'm going to offer you a compromise. Let's look at how "fast" or take-out foods can be more nutritious.

If you want a sandwich from the deli, avoid fatty meats and those mixed with mayonnaise and high-fat dressings. Instead, go for lean meats, veggies, and low-fat condiments such as mustards, pickle relishes, and tomato salsas. Add a salad to your meal. Skip heavy dressings, and try a little lemon juice and olive oil.

When searching out a hamburger, try to frequent a restaurant that grills meat rather than frying it. A grilled chicken breast sandwich piled high with fresh greens (without the mayonnaise) is also an option to consider. Pass on the fries, and experiment with baked potatoes stuffed with grilled veggies, herbs, yogurt, grated Parmesan cheese, or baked beans.

Most American Chinese food is full of fat. If you want Chinese take-out, try steamed noodle bowls with vegetables, tofu, or lean meats. Request steamed rice instead of fat-laden fried rice. Enjoy the tastes of freshly made (not fried) spring rolls, as opposed to deep-fried egg rolls. Pass on the peanut sauces, and go for light sweet-and-sour dips.

When most of us think of Mexican food, the next thought is fat, fat, and more fat. However, you *can* eat Mexican food if you follow a few simple rules. First, make sure your tortillas are not fried. Request fresh flour or corn tortillas. Replace fried beans, usually full of fat, with whole bean soups. Cheeses need to be served on the side so that you can limit your intake. Instead of enchiladas dripping in cheese and oil, order grilled fajitas. This dish consists of grilled meats or veggies rolled up in fresh flour tortillas, which are not fried. Cut down on the cheeses and sour cream, and pile on the salsa.

Take-out pastas are easy to find nowadays. When visiting your favorite Italian eatery, skip the pizza, and go for grilled veggies, lean meats, tomato sauces, and pastas. Add a green salad to complete the meal. Top off with oil-and-vinegar instead of typical "house" creamy Italian dressing.

Make sure you eat two nutritionally sound meals per day. At home, stock up on "grab foods," such as apples, oranges, bananas, carrot and celery sticks, dried fruit, whole-grain breads, low-fat crackers, fat-free granolas, and breakfast bars. Replace soda pop with herbal teas, juices, and mineral waters.

— **Supplement your take-out/grab-food diet.** If you're in relatively good health and are eating well, you might be able to get away with not taking supplements. As mentioned earlier, most divorcing people are under a great deal of stress, and they neglect their diets. Stress burns up stored vitamin and mineral reserves. If not replenished, the immune system will begin to suffer. This, in turn, leads to illness and depression. Taking a few supplements can remedy your problem. Your multivitamin does not have to be expensive or fancy. You'll want a multivitamin that contains all of the essential vitamins and minerals. In addition, stress supplements such as **zinc, Vitamin B complex,**

Vitamin C, and **free-form amino complex** should be considered. These supplements can be found at your local health food store and drugstore. Take as directed on the label. (**Note:** Never exceed 100 mg of zinc per day. Check your multivitamin before supplementing with this nutrient.)

A number of years ago, my poor stressed-out body needed a lot of help. I had worn myself down to a frazzle and needed a boost. So, I took off my vegetarian hat and turned to **raw adrenal** and **thymus glandular.** Taken as directed, these supplements give our own adrenal and thymus glands a hand in managing stress. So, give yourself and your body a break. Do what you can to keep nutritionally fit. Along with nutritional supplements, there are several herbs that have anti-stress characteristics.

— **De-stress with herbs. Schisandra** is an important herb for the Chinese herbalist. Long used as a tonic for stressful times, schisandra also supports those organs most affected by stress, such as the central nervous system, kidneys, and the adrenal glands. Another useful Chinese herb is **rehmanni.** This herb has been used as a longevity tonic for some time and is believed to have anti-stress benefits. Take either herb in capsule form as directed on the label. **Bilberry** is a wonderful restorative for the cells in our body. Stress causes cell destruction and mutation. This little herb can guard our cells against the damage of stress. (**Note:** Do not use bilberry leaves in tea form for more than three weeks.)

Ashwagandha, also known as **withania** and **Indian ginseng,** has long been used in Ayurvedic medicine for stress. Taken in capsule form, it's a wonderful corrective herb.

— **Take a bath.** When feeling overwhelmed with emotion and stress, treat yourself to an herbal bath with the essential oils of sweet **clary sage,** woodsy **juniper,** fresh **lavender,** lovely **ylang-ylang,** warm **nutmeg,** intoxicating **rosewood,** or reviving

orange. These scented oils can relax your whirling mind and settle the body. Lower your blood pressure with the music of crashing waves, a bubbling brook, bird calls, or seaside sounds.

— **Catnip** is a wonderful anti-stress herb. It's an easy plant to grow, and if taken as directed, it's very safe for human consumption. Not only does it calm the nervous system, but it can induce drowsiness. This is a great "unwind" herb. Take as directed on the label as a tea, glycerin tincture, or capsule.

— **Lemon balm** tea or glycerin tincture has traditionally been used to lift the spirits and reduce nervousness. Also, it's a useful remedy for heart palpitations.

— I can't say enough about **oats.** I use them in a glycerin tincture form during times of stress. This long-used remedy is safe, calming, not addictive, and nutritional.

— **Jujube,** another Chinese herbal remedy, not only increases stamina, but is mildly sedative.

— **Skullcap** is the nerveine (regulates the nervous system) for those of you to try who need a more potent herbal remedy for anxiety and stress. Use this herb in a tincture form with a glycerin base. Taken as directed, three times a day for a week, this funny-looking herb will restore your nervous system and reduce anxiety.
(**Note:** Do not use any of the above herbs if you're taking an antidepressant, tranquilizer, sleep medication, or muscle relaxers.)

Divorce is a life-changing event, with one door closing and many opening. When we end a relationship, we're confronted with several paths. We can quickly jump into another relationship and be at risk for repeating our mistakes; hide from life with work, our children, addictions, and isolation; or use this opportunity to make some positive life changes. Recovery from divorce is not an overnight experience, but a process that can take as long as several years. By putting one foot in front of the other and doing what is necessary to heal emotionally, physically, and spiritually, you will discover the wonder of *you.*

Eric knew he had to make some changes in his life. His wife, Marilyn, had left him for another man, and he had a lot of anger. Turning to his sister Pauline, he said, "I'm so angry with her. She really hurt me, and I can't run from it any longer. My rage is eating me up. I can't let this destroy me." While clearing the lunch plates from the table, Pauline stopped to give her brother a loving pat on the back. Eric gave her hand a squeeze and then turned his attention to his young nephew.

After putting the dishes in the sink, Pauline turned back to Eric and said, "You know, divorce doesn't have to be the end of your life. If you do what you need to do to heal, it can be a new beginning. Walk through the pain and rage, and you'll begin to see light at the end of this particular journey. I will be here for you."

Slowly, a tear slid down Eric's face. *No*, he thought, *I can't hide from this anymore.*

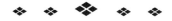

Chapter six

LET'S TALK ABOUT SEX

It was Friday afternoon, or "couples' day," as I like to call it. My husband and I have been seeing couples as a team for years. As therapists, we have found this particular mode of relationship therapy to be very effective. In our experience, one therapist with two people often sets off comments such as, "Well, the therapist is on *your* side; *I* didn't feel very supported."

The couple sitting on the couch was holding hands. Michael and I could both tell that they loved each other very much. Linda was brunette and feisty. She was eager to talk. Her husband, Glen, seemed more reserved. When doing relationship therapy, it's not uncommon for one partner to talk more than another.

"So, Linda," I began. "what made you decide to seek out marital therapy?"

Smoothing her skirt with well-manicured nails, Linda adjusted herself and then said, "We just aren't communicating." As she talked, I watched Glen zone out. He may have been sitting in our office, but his thoughts were elsewhere.

After Linda shared, Michael asked the two of them, "How is your sex life?" One of the things we, as helping professionals, have learned, is that couples rarely bring up the topic of sex, and if they do, this is done at the very end of the session. As such, we tend to ask about sex fairly early in the conversation.

Once again, Michael asked, "And how is sex?" Linda suddenly became quiet, and Glen's mind went off to another place again.

After a few moments of silence, I asked Glen, "How is your sexual relationship?" He was obviously embarrassed and uncomfortable. Linda was looking at her shoes while Glen picked his nails. Who would have thought that such a question would rattle two people who had been married for 25 years!

Finally, Glen took a deep breath, sighed, and said, "Well, actually that's what we really need to talk about." He then gave his wife a quick sideways glance. Linda had her legs and arms crossed. It was obvious that this was a difficult issue.

When we watch a lovemaking extravaganza on television or at the movies, everything seems so perfect. Romance oozes from every pore of the actors involved in the scene. The emotions are passionate, and the sex is explosive. Yes, the world of make-believe often leaves the rest of us feeling very inadequate. Why? Many of us use the image that the media portrays about relationships as a model for what our own intimate exchanges should look like. In today's society, we may see a lot of sex in popular culture, but most of us know very little about true intimacy.

Sexuality becomes even more confusing when we find that we're suddenly unable to perform sexually. For men, this is commonly referred to as impotence, while for women, a lack of sexual desire is seen as frigidity. Although these conditions can have true physical origins, many times they are psychological in nature. To date, the majority of sexual dysfunction cases we've seen in therapy have been tied to unresolved psychological issues.

(**Note:** If you're suffering from impotence or frigidity, I strongly suggest that you get a thorough physical by a qualified health-care provider before proceeding with options offered in this chapter. Underlying diseases, such as diabetes, high blood pressure, a history of sexually transmitted diseases, any circulatory impairment, paralysis, or atherosclerosis can contribute to impotence. Certain medications such as diuretics, antidepressants, sedatives, antihistamines, certain cholesterol-lowering drugs, antihypertensives, and, for men, antacids, can also disrupt sexual function. Hormonal imbalances and (as we shall see later) nutritional deficiencies can interfere with the sex drive in both men and women. If you're able to sexually arouse yourself with masturbation but find that you can't perform with your partner, your sexual difficulties are most likely psychological. Also, impotent men who are able to have erections during sleep are usually suffering from a psychological form of this disorder.

The Psychology of Sex

— **Confusing love with sex.** Love and sex are not the same thing. In a loving relationship, sex can be an expression of love. Sadly, in many relationships, sex is often used in a number of unloving ways. The act of sex can be used to temporarily "fix" a disagreement between two people. When this happens, the thought is, *If we have sex, this will smooth things out. How can we have a bad relationship if we're having sex?*

But having sex never resolves relationship problems. For the time being, it just sweeps them under the rug. Eventually they return.

Sex is also used as a weapon. "She cut her hair so I'm not going to have sex with her," or "He won't give me what I want. Why should I have sex with him?" Years ago, I was a guest on a TV talk show about men who wouldn't have sex with their wives because of weight gain. Yes, sex can be a powerful weapon. When sex is used as a method of control, this can lead to sexual dysfunction in one or both partners. When control and manipulation replace trust, care, and concern, sex is no longer a safe expression of love.

Take out a piece of paper and list how you have used the act of sex, a lack of sex, or sexual withdrawal as a means to control, punish, hurt, or to get what you want in a relationship. Next, list how your partner or past partners have used sex to control or manipulate you. Finally, write a short letter to your partner about how you honestly feel about your sex life. List what you like and dislike about your sexual encounters. Before giving this note to your mate, share it with a therapist, spiritual advisor, or health-care practitioner. If necessary, read this letter to your partner while in the company of a third party.

— **Old history and past relationships.** For years, I've worked with men and women who have had sexual difficulties. Many of these issues are the result of some form of sexual violation experienced in youth or in adulthood. When most of us think about sexual violation, we immediately focus on penetration. This tends to be society's definition of sexual violation. Sexual abuse comes in many shapes and forms, and it isn't always intentional. Whenever touch feels wrong, it probably *is* wrong. Inappropriate sexual touch can affect sexual performance and intimacy.

Many types of abuse are by-products of parents or caretakers who don't know how to educate their children about sex. This is called "unintentional abuse." The following scenarios are a by-product of caretakers "not knowing any better." It's important to understand that this type of abuse is not intentional. Check the following as they apply to your history:

- Got inadequate information about human sexuality, puberty, sexual function, and menstruation while growing up.

- Was given false information from caregivers while growing up, such as, "If you masturbate, your penis will fall off," "Nice girls don't like sex," "Sex is dirty," and "Sex is only for procreation."
- Received too much information about sex at too early an age.
- Had no privacy in the bathroom as a child. Had no sexual boundaries in the home. Caregivers didn't lock doors during sex when children were around.
- Experienced sexually repressed (or overtly sexual) caregivers. Rarely saw parents hug or kiss one another. A test: Even now, can you imagine your parents having sex?
- Was reprimanded for sexual behavior with threats of retribution by God or religion, such as "God will punish you for masturbating" or "Sex before a marriage is sin." Told that those who have homosexual or lesbian relationships were "going to hell."
- Often overheard comments or jokes that were extremely sexual in nature.
- Was shown pornographic material as a child.
- Was often in the vicinity of adults who were not cautious around children with respect to dress or bathroom behavior, especially during adolescence. On the extreme end of this continuum would be exposure to those with over cautious behavior with regard to nudity or bathroom activity.
- Had parents who talked about their issues in front of the children.
- Was exposed to the extramarital affairs of caretakers. This indirectly impacts children's sexual development,

even if the affair is a secret. Such secrets create intimacy issues for future generations.

- Experienced the excessive use of enemas or medical procedures involving the sex organs.

- Had parents or caregivers who were sexually abused themselves. These individuals often have difficulty passing on healthy sexuality to their children.

The previous incidents are very common and are often at the core of sexual difficulties. A good therapist or spiritual advisor can assist you in working through these old issues. In addition, I strongly suggest that you get some appropriate information on human sexuality. The following incidents are considered direct, intentional acts of sexual violation. These types of violations can come from a variety of sources—such as strangers, relatives, teachers, co-workers, scout leaders, clergy, siblings, and, yes, even past or present partners.

- Being called a slut, whore, gigolo, or other degrading name, at any age.

- Being subjected to unwanted back rubs, massages, hand-holding, hugging, touching, dancing, or kissing, at any age.

- Experiencing breast or genital touching or fondling by an adult in childhood or as an adult. Experiencing rape, at any age.

- Being forced to be masturbated or to masturbate another, at any age.

- Experiencing, in childhood, penetration—genitally, anal, or orally—with fingers, objects, or sexual organs by anyone who is older or bigger.

- In adulthood, experiencing genital, anal, or oral penetration with fingers, objects, or sexual organs by anyone (including a primary partner, husband, wife, lover) by force.

- Being exposed to the genitals of a "flasher."

- Being forced to watch another person being sexually assaulted, at any age.

The above examples of sexual assault are only a few of those on a list I use with clients. These experiences can dramatically impact sexual relations and performance in adulthood. If you've checked off any of these, you might want to take some time to explore how these incidents are affecting your sexuality today. Refer to Chapter 7 for more information on how to work through such violations. If you need help, don't hesitate to seek out a health-care provider who understands sexual issues. At this point, it's also important to recognize that depression, rage, and extreme fear are normal reactions to sexual violation. If these emotions were not processed at the time of the trauma, they can greatly contribute to sexual dysfunction in the future. For information on effectively addressing these strong emotions, refer to Chapter 3 for rage recovery, Chapter 2 for resolution of depression, and Chapter 9 to heal from fear. Separating past sexual history from current relationships enables us to begin experiencing the joy of healthy intimacy.

Lifestyle Remedies for Healthy Sex

— **Stress reduction.** There are many different types of stress, and each of these can create sexual difficulties. As we've seen above, unresolved psychological stress resulting from trauma will interfere with healthy, loving sexual function. Let's look at some other types of stress that can be equally damaging.

Current worries over finances, employment, marital problems, family difficulties, and job dissatisfaction can manifest as sexual difficulty. Good sex requires a state of relaxation. If we're distracted with other concerns, the act of sex can feel like one more pressure.

Sexual failure, the inability to perform, or a lack of desire creates stress. When intimacy is initiated by your partner, do you feel pressure to perform? Such stress can compound impotence or frigidity, making lovemaking even more difficult.

Unresolved relationship issues create distance and distrust between couples. It's difficult to let go sexually if lack of trust is an issue. When we experience orgasm, we are at our most vulnerable. How can we allow ourselves to be vulnerable if we can't trust our partner? Do *you* trust your sex partner? If not, list why, and share this with a trusted confidant.

Take out another piece of paper and list all of the types of stress you're currently experiencing. You may need some help in sorting these out, too. If you do, visit with a therapist, spiritual advisor, trusted friend, or support group.

— **Get back in touch with your body.** Healthy touch often helps us get back in touch with our bodies. Massages, facials, and reflexology can assist in reconnecting to our physical selves. Another way to nurture the body is with self-massage during a bath. One woman I worked with suffered from severe frigidity. Every time she and her husband attempted to have intercourse, her vaginal area would tighten up. This left her frustrated, depressed, and miserable. In her younger years, she had been raped by a boyfriend. After guided visualization therapy, she discovered that every time she attempted to have intercourse with her husband, her emotions were being triggered, and her body "remembered" the rape. Sex for this woman was both physically and emotionally painful.

In another case I worked on, a young man would lose his erection each time he tried to engage in intercourse. In this instance, his body was also remembering sexual abuse. This trauma involved a violation to his penis by a neighbor during childhood. Sexual intercourse flooded him with memories of this act.

Once these traumas were emotionally processed, I suggested to each of these individuals that they attempt self-massage, which involves gently touching the part of the body that is not responding normally to sexual arousal. While doing so, an affirmation is repeated. "You are perfect, safe, and I love you." For both clients, the experience was very emotional and healing. The body will remember past trauma, and situations in the here-and-now can trigger the feelings of such experiences.

— **Do what works.** Returning to the media once again, many of us believe that our sexual experiences must look like those on TV or in the movies. According to Hollywood, flames of passion need to be erupting as we gasp for breath in between suffocating kisses. If sexual dysfunction is an issue, such smoldering love scenes can make one feel extremely inadequate.

I have a simple remedy for this problem. First, we must never compare our lovemaking abilities with those presented to us by the media. Second, if some type of sexual activity doesn't feel right, make a change. I'm an incest survivor, and a great deal of my abuse took place on a bed. When I began working on this issue, I found that I would freeze up every time Michael and I became sexually intimate in our bed. The solution to this was quite simple. For a period of time, the bedroom was off limits, but other areas of the house were fair game.

If one form of sexual acting-out creates difficulty, try something else. Don't push yourself to participate in a particular sexual act if it creates problems for you. If you do force yourself to attempt to perform, you will end up resenting your partner and feeling uncomfortable about sex. If you don't feel safe during the act of sex, turn on the lights, keep a favorite blanket with you for comfort, or ask your partner to climb into a bubble bath with you. When an attempt at intercourse leaves you feeling impotent and miserable, use masturbation with your partner. Experiment with lotions, body creams, or oils. If oral sex is difficult, try something else. Play with scented soaps and have sex in the shower. In other words, don't do the same thing over and over again if it isn't working. Try something different.

— **Make time for intimate, uninterrupted sex.** Need I say more? Once we really take the time to examine the psychological issues that have set up the sexual dysfunction, we can begin to implement the lifestyle changes that will return us to healthy sexual functioning. Certain nutritional changes and herbal remedies can also give us an added push toward creating the healthy sense of sexuality we all deserve.

Nutrition and Herbs for a Healthy Sex Life

Diet plays an important role in healthy sexual function. In order to assure that hormone levels are balanced, the blood system is flowing properly, and nerve function is up to par, it's essential that we take care in choosing what we put in our bodies. In working with people who have food addictions, I have heard that it's not uncommon for the sufferers of anorexia nervosa, bulimia, or compulsive eating to have low sex drives. What this tells me is that a good diet is needed to promote physical health. When we have optimal physical health, we will have a healthy sex drive.

— **What to eat.** A diet high in grains, complex carbohydrates, vegetables, lean meats, or vegetable protein such as soy, fish, and fruit will keep the blood flowing and the body healthy. A diet high in saturated fats not only clogs the blood vessels around the heart, but it can also interfere with blood flow to the penis. Imagine that! If the small blood vessels in the penis are not clear, this can interfere with sexual response. Nicotine also causes these blood vessels to constrict. For both men and women, excessive use of alcohol will also impair sexual function.

— Nutritional supplementation for frigidity and impotency. As we've seen, the inability for men (impotence) and women to enjoy sex (frigidity) is often the result of a past sexual trauma. Although this is usually the case, this condition can be a by-product of nutritional deficiencies. For women, such shortages can affect estrogen production. Too little estrogen can create a lack of lubrication, making intercourse painful. In rare instances, a deficiency in testosterone can create impotence in men. These conditions can be corrected with proper nutrition, herbal remedies, and, if needed, hormonal supplementation. Both sexes should consider taking a good multivitamin and mineral supplement. A woman's nutritional supplement program should also include 500 IUs of **Vitamin E** per day. Increase this to 1,500 IUs per day over time. Men need to increase their intake of Vitamin E to at least 1,000 mg. Vitamin E is also known as a sex vitamin because it assists the reproductive system and the functioning of the glands.

(**Note:** If you have high blood pressure or are on an anticoagulant medication, check with your health-care provider before using this supplement.)

Vitamin C intake needs to be increased to 5,000 mg per day. Divide this into 2–3 doses. This nutrient is essential for proper glandular function. **Zinc** appears to play an important role in healthy sexual function in both men and women. A deficiency in this mineral can disrupt sexual function in women. For men, a lack of zinc interferes not only with the production of testosterone, but with the health of the prostate. Women and men should supplement their diet with approximately 50 mg of zinc per day.

(**Note:** Your total intake of this nutrient should never be more than 100 mg per day.)

Now that we've looked at vitamin/mineral supplements, let's see what herbal remedies are useful for sexual difficulties.

— **Damiana** has testosterogenic properties and is believed to be useful in restoring sexuality in both men an women. This traditional Mayan aphrodisiac should be used as directed in tablet or tincture form. **Muira puama** will also stimulate the libido. Other aphrodisiacs are **jasmine** and **ylang-ylang**.

(**Note:** Do not use the essential oil of ylang-ylang internally.)

— **Chinese ginseng,** the most famous of all Chinese herbs, is a useful remedy for men and women. Because this herb contains constituents that the body can use to make sex hormones, herbalists continue to suggest Chinese ginseng for improving sexual function. Choose a standardized extract in capsule form, and take half of the dose directed on the label for several weeks. Then, increase this to a full dose.

(**Note:** Do not use this herb if you have high blood pressure, are sensitive to stimulants, or suffer from hypoglycemia or heart disease.)

— **Schisandra** is another well-known Chinese herb that can be used to increase sexual desire in both men and women. Not only will it increase sexual stamina, but it also improves the secretion of the sex fluids. This herb can be difficult to find, but be persistent. Look for it in capsule form, and take as directed on the label. **Yohimbe** also improves blood flow to the sexual organs. (**Note:** Use this herb only under the supervision of a knowledgeable health-care provider.)

— The essential oils **patchouli** and **sandalwood** have long been used to heighten sexual desire. Invite your sex partner to climb into a warm bath scented with these two exotic oils and see what happens. If that doesn't work, try a massage. Put several drops of patchouli and sandalwood oil into almond oil, and gently rub this into your mate's skin.

All of us deserve a healthy sex life. If we are willing to clean up any past psychological sex-related traumas, we have a good chance of reclaiming our sexual selves. In addition, we must examine how our lifestyle and diet might be complicating this part of our lives. As we have seen, hormonal imbalances and illnesses can also be at the core of sexual dysfunction. If this is the case, these conditions must be remedied before addressing sexual issues.

The therapy session was almost over. Michael and I had determined that the couple had not had a sexual encounter for months. In spite of this fact, they wanted to focus on a number of other issues. "Okay. We all know there's a sex problem, and for the last 40 minutes we've talked about everything but sex." There was silence. It was obvious to me that it was time to pull out the big guns.

"Do you know that in this country, it's estimated that approximately 30 million men suffer from some type of impotence at one time or another? And are you aware that periodic frigidity among women is extremely common?" As I said these words, Linda and Glen looked extremely surprised.

"So," I asked, " who wants to go first?"

The two of them looked at one another, and then in unison, said, "I will."

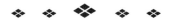

*C*hapter seven

ABUSIVE RELATIONSHIPS: THERE IS HOPE

Lydia ran to the small downstairs bathroom and locked the door. Crying hysterically, she then moved the clothes hamper up against the door. Suddenly, Larry was beating on the door and yelling at the top of his lungs.

"Lydia! You come out here right now! We aren't done discussing this!" Sobbing, Lydia continued to push all of her weight against the wooden hamper. She had been through this before and knew that her husband's rages could escalate into physical mistreatment. Three months ago, she was carrying a stick of thick pancake makeup in her pocket at all times. Lydia thanked God for this makeup, because it usually did a great job of covering up little bruises.

Unfortunately, after their last argument two weeks ago, the makeup was of little use. Larry had violently pushed her to the floor, and she had hit the side of her head on the leg of a coffee table. Lydia hated lying to the children, her family, and friends about the huge black-and-blue mark on her face. This go-around, she was determined not to let that happen again. Little bruises were one thing, but the big ones were just too hard to hide.

"Lydia," cried Larry, "I just want to talk to you! I'm sorry I frightened you. Can we please just talk?" Larry slumped to the ground on the other side of the door. He then cradled his head in his hands. "Honey," he said softly, "I'm sorry I called you all of those awful names."

On the other side of the bathroom door, Lydia was whimpering and shaking with fear. *I love him so much,* she thought to herself, *but I can't keep putting up with this! Yeah, now he's beginning to feel guilty for screaming at me and calling me every dirty, rotten name in the book. Tomorrow he'll buy me a beautiful bouquet of flowers or a piece of expensive jewelry. I know this routine.* Slowly, Lydia reached for a bit of toilet tissue and began wiping away the dark, running eye makeup and tears. "In a month," she cried softly to herself, "he'll get angry with me over some small, insignificant thing and then erupt again. I just don't know what to do!"

According to U.S. Department of Justice statistics, more than half a million women a year experience violent victimization by husbands and boyfriends. Women are not the only ones who are victimized by abuse. Every day, children and even men experience emotional, physical, and sexual violation. Why do those who are being abused in a relationship have such a difficult time leaving such a situation? I've worked with abused adults and children for more than two decades, so let me share with you what I've learned.

The Psychology of Abusive Relationships

— **The protection of dissociation.** Years ago I was on a national TV talk show discussing domestic violence. As the "expert," it was my job to explain to the audience why women and men stay with abusive partners. Sitting with me was a woman who had endured a great deal of both emotional and physical mistreatment by her husband. Half of the studio audience was loudly chastising the woman. This made it almost impossible for me to offer my opinion on the topic. Comments such as, "What's wrong with you?" "Are you insane?" "Stupid!" "How could you stay in that relationship for so long?" "Why did you let him hit you in front of your children?" and "You are a failure as a mother," flew at this poor woman. As the crowd continued to berate her, I watched her eyes glaze over as she shut down both emotionally and physically. To survive the abuse of the audience, she did what she had done so often to withstand the trauma of her relationship: She dissociated herself from the people abusing her.

If you're in a relationship with a partner who regularly abuses you verbally or physically, and you're having a difficult time leaving this situation, let me offer you an explanation for your behavior. Interestingly, my own family history provides the perfect backdrop.

My father verbally and physically abused my mother. He was very unhappy with himself and had difficulty handling his anger. This set the stage for many violent outbursts. With each round of harsh, verbal treatment, my frightened mother would ask herself, "What did I do?" In other words, she would exchange a healthy reality that said, "This is hurtful and wrong," for very unhealthy reasoning, such as, "Maybe this is my fault and I deserve his rage." On other occasions, she would say to herself, "He doesn't really mean what he says. He's just tired." This is how my mother survived. By accepting my father's reasoning and by finding excuses for his behavior, she was able to endure his abusive words. Eventually, for my mother, this form of emotional dissociation became an automatic response to my father's intimidating and frightening rages.

When my father began physically assaulting my mother, a new form of dissociation took over. Whereas before, she could dissociate emotionally from the abuse with minimization, rationalization, excuses, and denial, she now needed to learn how to physically shut down. Women, men, and children who are physically abused learn to distance themselves from their physical bodies when they're being physically hurt. How often I have heard, "I was going to show him. I wasn't about to cry," or "I'm so used to it. It doesn't even register with me anymore. It always passes." Does this mean that the shove, slap, or violent beating doesn't hurt? Absolutely not. Individuals who are confronted with abuse learn how to "survive" it by ignoring the hurt. Sadly, this is also how severe injury and even death can occur. Physical pain alerts us to a problem with the body. Abuse survivors learn to ignore this warning sign.

As a result of both witnessing and experiencing abuse, I was very at-risk for an abusive marriage myself. Before I could have a successful relationship with another person, I needed to investigate several notions about abuse:

- Dissociation saved me as a child, but would hurt me as an adult. I needed to begin to listen to my emotional and physical pain. Ignoring this problem was no longer a solution.

- I had to recognize that abuse was not a normal by-product of a relationship. Excessive name-calling, raging, shaming, belittling, and cursing is abusive and hurtful. Physical violence, be it pushing, hitting, biting, throwing things, or violent sexual attacks do not belong in a loving partnership.

- If I stay in an abusive relationship, not only am I hurting myself, but I'm hurting my partner. As long as I allow my partner to hurt me, this individual will never take responsibility for his inappropriate behavior. If this person is never held accountable for his actions, he will not be able to heal.

- By allowing myself to be emotionally controlled, abused, physically restrained, shoved, injured, or sexually hurt, I am passing on a message to my children that says, "This is acceptable behavior."

If you're in an emotionally, physically, or even sexually abusive relationship, take out a piece of paper and write down how you're doing the following:

- Dissociating from the abuse—minimizing, rationalizing and excusing harsh words or hurtful touch.
- Accepting the abuse.
- Avoiding growth—not evolving into the creative, spiritual being you deserve to be.
- Permitting the abuse to continue, and keeping your partner from healing as a result.
- Allowing the abuse to impact any children you may have. What messages are you passing on to your children by not taking a stand, getting help, or leaving the situation?

Today I'm not in an abusive relationship, but this never would have happened if I hadn't looked closely at the above questions.

Lifestyle Remedies for Healing from Abusive Relationships

— **Do I have to leave?"** This is a question that I'm often asked by those who are experiencing abuse by their partners. Do you have to leave when abuse is taking place? Yes. This is the goal of your healing. Do you have to divorce or separate from your abusing partner? Not necessarily. If you're willing to make the lifestyle changes required for your healing, you just might have a chance with this partner. Write a short essay on why it's difficult for you to leave the scene when you're being emotionally, physically, or sexually mistreated.

— **Understanding the inability to leave.** At one time, I was in an emotionally abusive relationship. My partner would criticize me, put me down, and belittle me. When such abuse would start, I became frozen, powerless, and felt I did not have a choice when it came to leaving. Eventually I discovered I *did* have an option. The following visualization helped me sort out why leaving was so difficult:

> *Find a quiet place where you can be alone. Close your eyes and visualize yourself at many different ages, such as 3, 5, 10, 13, 16, 20, 25, and older. Imagine all of those individuals of different ages sitting together playing a game. See yourself as you are today, walking into this scene, and then ask, "Which one of you is frightened of my [husband, boyfriend, wife, girlfriend, partner, friend, or lover]? Why do you think I continue to put up with this?" Listen closely, and see if anyone answers. Once you've identified those who are frightened of your partner, tell them that you're going to learn how to remove yourself from abusive situations. Upon hearing this, see if any of these inner you's are relieved. Finally, tell them that none of them deserve the mistreatment all of you are receiving. Open your eyes and write down your experience. Share this with a therapist, spiritual advisor, or friend.*

— **Making a plan of action to leave when it's necessary.** Write out a plan for removing yourself from future, unhealthy situations. Have a spare set of keys to your car made and put them in a secret place in the garage. Next, pack a bit of cash with some toiletries, a set of nightclothes, and undergarments in a small duffel bag. Hide this as well. Third, ask close friends if, on the spur of the moment, you can come and stay with them. The next time that your partner emotionally, physically, or sexually hurts you, wait until he or she has fallen asleep and then *leave*. After being away for three days, telephone, but don't tell your partner where you are. Instead, let your partner know that he must commit to getting help before you're willing to come back.

In working with those caught up in an abusive relationship, I always tell them that if their partner is willing to seek out assistance for their behavior, the relationship has a good chance of surviving. As long as ill-treated individuals continue to allow themselves to be harmed, their partners will never look for solutions to their explosive or controlling behavior. Breaking this type of cycle can only happen if you refuse to enable your mate's inappropriate conduct. As long as you put up with this type of destructive acting-out, you're enabling the relationship to stay dysfunctional. If you have children, be sure to include them in your plan. Many individuals have difficulty putting such a plan together, so if this is the case, don't hesitate to reach out for help.

(**Note:** When things are running smoothly in your relationship, enjoy this time. If the tone of the relationship turns dark, frightening, and unpredictable, take a time-out.)

— **Try positive affirmations.** Those of us who stay with an abusive partner usually have low self-esteem. If we had a positive sense of self-worth, we would have done something about this abuse ages ago. Nobody can increase our self-esteem except us. Take out three small pieces of paper, and on each piece, write:

- I deserve respect, not abuse, from every person in my life.

- I love myself enough to want to protect myself from the hurtful actions of others.

- I have a right to exist and be happy.

- I matter to the Universe.

Put one piece of paper on the dashboard of your car, the second in your wallet, and the third on the mirror in your bathroom.

Nutrition and Herbs for Recovery from Abusive Relationships

— **Let's keep it simple.** Because self-esteem often suffers when one is in a dysfunctional relationship, nutritional self-care isn't usually a top priority. Meals are skipped; fast foods fill in for homemade, nutritious dishes; and stimulants such as coffee or diet colas replace life-giving spring waters, herbal teas, or fresh juices. Understanding this, it's essential that the initial steps for improving your nutritional state be kept simple. I want you to succeed. If I complicate the cornflakes with too many nutritional changes, chances are that this plan could be just a bit too overwhelming. I will keep these nutritional suggestions to a minimum, but understand that all of these bare essentials must be followed.

Before we look at dietary changes, let's do a little "mind work." Take three pieces of paper and write:

- I deserve nutritional health.

- My nutritional health improves my state of mind.

- With physical and emotional well-being, I can make healthy decisions that are in my best interest.

Put one note on your refrigerator, a second in your wallet, and the third on the dashboard of your car. These little notes will remind you to take care of your nutritional needs.

— Supplement once a day to counter "fight-or-flight" stress reaction. The fight-or-flight reaction occurs when we are under extreme stress and/or are feeling threatened. Confronting emotional, physical, or sexual mistreatment places tremendous hardship on the body. When your partner is hurting you, your heartbeat increases and your blood pressure soars. In addition, your metabolic rate shoots up. These increases are a by-product of the hormones called adrenaline and cortisol.

Living in an abusive relationship leaves you in a constant state of anxiety. These stressful physical and emotional states deplete the body of nutrients. As a result, it's absolutely necessary for you to take a potent daily multivitamin and mineral supplement. This supplement must give you more than the recommended daily allowance (RDA) for vitamins and minerals. Ask the health-store clerk to show you a multivitamin and mineral formula that:

- is specifically for those living a stressful lifestyle, and
- needs to be taken only once a day.

That's right. Only one dose of vitamins per day. I told you we were going to keep it simple. This one nutritional suggestion will do your body a world of good.

— Cut down on caffeine and alcohol. Both of these substances add stress to the body. Alcohol depresses your central nervous system, while caffeine pumps it up. If you want to relax, there are numerous herbal teas that will do the trick. (Read the next section on herbs for information on relaxing herbal teas.) Also, switch to a decaffeinated coffee.

— **The Caveman Diet.** I love the Caveman Diet and use it when I'm under a great deal of stress. The Caveman Diet consists of numerous healthy "grab foods." These nutritious eats replace processed, fatty cookies, crackers, candies, and fast foods. Not only will this diet work for you, but it can improve your entire family's eating habits. What does the Caveman Diet consist of?

Let's begin with soy products. In recent years, soy milks have become very popular. They can be found at grocery and health food stores, in individual and large serving sizes. Soy milk contains isoflavones that help reduce cholesterol and may assist in building bone density. Stress can actually increase cholesterol levels. Be good to yourself, and instead of that cola, cut cholesterol with a glass of chocolate or vanilla soy milk.

Soy nuts come in a variety of flavors, such as garlic, barbecue, and honey roasted. I throw a handful of these tasty nuts in my salad, and carry a small bag of them in my purse. These tasty treats make for a quick "pick-me-up."

Clean the junk foods out of your cupboards, and replace them with dry-roasted almonds, granolas sweetened with fruit juices, dried raisins, and fruits. Whole-grain breads or rye crackers provide a good base for a sandwich made of low-fat cheeses, lean meats, or protein-filled nut butters. In the refrigerator, store celery and carrot sticks. These prepared vegetables can be found in the produce section of most grocery stores and go well with nutritious tofu or low-fat yogurt dips. As a matter of fact, nowadays, **Vitamin A**-rich carrot sticks can be found in individual serving packs. On your kitchen counters, fill bowls with a variety of fruits for mid-morning or afternoon snacks.

Natural fruit juices, bottled water, and herbal teas need to replace coffee and cola drinks. You can find a variety of herbal fruit tea bags at your health-food or grocery store. Throw a couple of herbal tea bags in a pitcher of hot water from the tap, and let this sit for several hours. Green tea is also a wonderful option for the serious coffee drinker. Not only has green tea been shown to have cancer-preventing properties, but its caffeine content is much lower than regular coffees and teas.

If you want to sweeten your tea, avoid using sugar. Table sugar not only increases the excretion of valuable minerals and vitamins from your body, but it also disrupts blood-sugar levels and decreases the immune system's ability to fight off disease and illness. Sweeten your tea with **stevia**, a natural sweetener made from stevia leaves. Stevia (*Stevia rebaudiana bertoni*) is much sweeter than pure table sugar, so you don't have to use that much of it.

All of the above Caveman Diet suggestions can be utilized by just about anyone, and they require little, if any, preparation. Take an hour a week to stock your cupboards and refrigerator with these yummy edibles. Once you have done so, you'll be able to "grab," when needed, an assortment of nutritious foods for your body. By properly feeding yourself and taking one multivitamin and mineral supplement per day, your self-esteem will improve by leaps and bounds.

Now it's time to investigate a few of the herbal remedies that can improve the state of your emotional, physical, and spiritual well-being:

— **Nutritional help from the plant world.** When I'm working with an individual who's caught up in an abusive relationship, his or her nutritional state is of primary concern. I believe that emotional stress leads to nutritional deficiencies. A poorly fed body is a breeding ground for cancer, heart disease, high blood pressure, hypoglycemia, high cholesterol, gall bladder problems, diabetes, and a host of other illnesses. Along with the above nutritional guidelines, let me offer two other suggestions. **Bee pollen** is full of necessary nutrients. This powdery substance is collected from flowers by bees and can assist in strengthening the immune system. Because of its protein, vitamin, and mineral content, bee pollen is also useful in fighting fatigue and depression. This supplement can be found at most health food stores and should be taken as directed.

(**Note:** A very small number of people are allergic to bee pollen. Start out with a small dose, and if you find that you're suddenly coughing, wheezing, developing a rash, or experiencing other symptoms, stop using it.)

Spirulina, the "green food" of the new millennium, contains an enormous amount of plant protein and is especially useful for the individual experiencing a great deal of stress. Not only is it packed full of essential vitamins and minerals, it's easy to digest, protects the immune system, controls blood-sugar levels, checks cholesterol, and encourages the absorption of minerals. Spirulina should be purchased in tablet form.

— **A little bit more about stress reduction. Suma tea** has a rich, hearty flavor, and it's a great coffee substitute. Also referred to as **Brazilian ginseng,** suma tea is an incredible immune-system booster. In addition, it wards off anemia and fights stress and fatigue. If I'm burning the candle at both ends, you can bet I'll be drinking large quantities of suma tea. Suma teabags can be found at your health food store.

Bach Rescue Remedy is another source of relief. This tincture of flower essence works similar to that of a homeopathic remedy. When you're feeling overwhelmed, hopeless, and stressed to the max, add four drops of Rescue Remedy to a cup of **chamomile, red clover,** or **balm tea.**

— **Speaking of herbal teas.** Often the emotional stress of a dysfunctional relationship can leave us feeling very blue, indeed. This depressed state makes decision-making even more difficult. If you're feeling beaten down by life, try using the following herbal remedies: **Vervain** was used by the Pawnee Indians to heighten their dream states and has a long history of use as a mood enhancer. Steep vervain with peppermint or lemon balm tea, and keep refrigerated for those stressful moments. **Wild lettuce** was once called "lettuce opium" because of its ability to calm an excited state of mind. This herb is recognized by the German government as an appropriate treatment for depression and nervousness. Wild lettuce tea bags can be carried in the wallet or purse and should be used when anxiety strikes.

— **The scents of nature.** Before we end this chapter, I would like to discuss how aromatherapy can be used to correct a hopeless state of mind. A whiff of the essential oils of certain herbs can do much to change our perceptions of the world. Years ago, I was going through a particularly rough time. When feeling overwhelmed, I would pull out a vial of the essential oils **patchouli, jasmine,** or **sandalwood.** One sniff usually did the trick.

On my back porch, the scent of a patchouli plant fills the air. The essential oil of this herb has a calming effect on the mind, and I often sit on my porch just to breathe in this scent. Sandalwood is another one of my all-time favorite fragrances. Used in China for thousands of years, this oil can help combat melancholia. Speaking of mood-enhancing scents, have you ever had a cup of jasmine tea at a Chinese restaurant? Also known as the "king of flowers," the scent of jasmine will chase fear away.

If you're having a particularly tough day, take a time-out. Brew up a cup of jasmine tea, dab a bit of patchouli or sandalwood oil on a tissue, find a quiet place to sit, and then breathe in the rich, soothing aroma of these herbs.

Living within an abusive relationship is extremely difficult. Getting out of such a toxic environment can prove to be even more troublesome. If you're being seriously injured, physically or sexually, I need to tell you that your plight will not improve. It may be necessary for you to leave the relationship for several days to gather your thoughts, clear your mind, and make healthy decisions. If you decide to stay in this relationship, you will need to develop behaviors that will allow you to take care of yourself. Enabling abusive behavior from a mate is not in your partner's best interest, and it will certainly not do you any good. If you need some assistance in learning how to protect yourself from emotional, physical, or sexual abuse, call your local United Way agency or family service center. Don't live your life as my mother did. Break out of the cycle of trauma by learning how to love yourself.

"What is that wonderful smell?" Lydia asked. She was having lunch with her sister Jill.

As she took a bite of her spinach salad, Jill answered, "That's my power scent. I take the essential oils of orange, coriander, and rose, and mix them with a bit of almond oil." Jill then held out her wrist so that her sister could smell the delightful perfume she had created for herself. "The scent of this particular combination of oils gives me courage."

After breathing in the rich smell of her sister's oils, Lydia stopped eating, and for a moment, became silent. She then looked off into the distance and murmured, "I could sure use some courage."

Jill suddenly put her fork down. "Lydia, this has gone on for too long. The whole family knows you're miserable!"

Stunned, Lydia turned to her sister. "What are you talking about? I'm not miserable!"

Jill then became very upset and said, "Do you think we don't know how he treats you? Lately it's all we talk about."

With this, Lydia began to cry, "But I love him. I don't want to leave him!"

Jill moved her chair closer to her sister's and said, "Honey, I'm not telling you to leave him, but I want you to get some help. You don't have to do this all by yourself. I will be here for you, but you need more than I can give. You may not know this, but years ago, Pete and I had an awful relationship."

Lydia wiped her eyes with her napkin and replied, "Really? What did you do about it?"

As she patted her sister on the back, Jill answered, "I learned how to respect, love, and take care of myself. Once I did this, Pete had two options. He could either grow with me, or go. I'm thankful he chose to grow, but I don't think that ever would have happened if I hadn't taken the first step. When will *you* take the first step?"

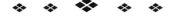

PART III

Do Control Issues Control You?

❧ ❧ ❧ ❧

Chapter eight

PANIC ATTACKS: SECRET PROTECTORS

Suzy climbed into the front seat of her father's huge gray Buick. The family was getting together for Thanksgiving at her sister's house, and she was dreading it. Suzy had recently filed for divorce from her alcoholic husband, and her family was not very happy about this state of affairs. While buckling her seat belt, she thought, *They treat me like an idiot, and act as if I'm some half-wit teenager who can't think for herself.*

As the car pulled on to the main street, Suzy's father asked, "Have you heard from Stanley lately?" Upon hearing her ex's name, she felt her blood pressure rise. *Why does he have to do this?* Suzy silently raged. *Pressure, pressure, pressure! Can't he just let me be? Why can't he understand I don't want to talk with Stanley!*

"No, Daddy," she replied. "I haven't heard from Stanley, and I really don't want to talk about him right now."

With this, her father shook his head in disapproval and then added, "We need to swing by your brother's house and pick him up." As he buzzed through a yellow light, Suzy's heart started to pound, and she could feel her blood pressure rise. She thought about her brother and ex-husband meeting two to three times a week to drink at their favorite bar. When Suzy filed for divorce, her brother had sided with Stanley .

"Will you slow down, please? Your driving really frightens me," she said as her father screeched into Jim's driveway.

While they waited for Jim, her father added, "Suzy, you really need to lighten up on Stanley. He's a good guy. You should give him another chance."

Sweat was now dripping down her back, and she felt as if she were having a heart attack. Gulping her breath, Suzy could feel her throat constricting. Grabbing the handle to the car door, Suzy cried, "Daddy, I just have to get out of this car!"

The Psychology of Panic Attacks

Just about everyone has experienced that momentary sense of panic. Before taking a test at school, going on a blind date, meeting a new person, confronting a difficult situation, or upon hearing bad news, the adrenaline rush of sudden panic can create the physical sensation of the "fight-or-flight" response. When this happens, the body responds with muscle tension, and an increase in heart rate and breathing. The physical body is preparing for a high-stress situation.

Several winters ago, I was skiing in Taos, New Mexico, with my family. It was the end of a glorious day, and we were riding down the mountain in the back of a cart being pulled by a truck. The cart was taking us down from the ski area to the parking lot below. Suddenly, I heard a very loud "thump." Looking behind me, I spotted a body crumpled up on the roadway. Immediately, my heart began to pound as the adrenaline quickly flowed through my veins. Jumping off the cart, I broke into a full run and dashed to the side of a man lying in the snow and mud. Looking into his eyes, it was apparent that he was moving in and out of consciousness, so I quickly did what was necessary to ensure his safely. At that moment in time, I needed a physical rush of adrenaline to assist me in this particular situation. My physical reactions allowed me to take immediate action in helping the injured man.

But what about Suzy? Why was *her* body responding in the "fight-or-flight" mode? There was no immediate physical danger in her environment. Why was she in the throes of a serious panic attack?

— **The loss of control.** For those suffering from panic attacks, it's important to know that environmental stimuli in the here-and-now can trigger these attacks. For each person afflicted with panic attacks, the stimuli or triggers are different. The length and intensity of panic attacks also varies for each sufferer. Many individuals have attacks during the day, while others only experience them at night. For some sufferers, there can be a sense of impending doom, death, and destruction. Others find that such attacks cause the mind to fog, and decision making becomes an impossibility. Numerous people experience these attacks on a periodic basis, while others are plagued with weekly or even daily panic attacks.

Although panic attacks are different for everyone, they do have one thing in common: Panic attacks function as marvelous survival skills. Yes, there is a reason for their existence, and as long as it's needed, the condition will remain. Confused? Let's return to Suzy for clarification in this matter.

Suzy tended to have panic attacks when she was around certain members of her family. Although she didn't start having these attacks until she was in her mid-20s, this behavior can occur at any stage of life and usually does so in response to specific life situations. Poor Suzy had a hard time standing up to both her brother and her father. Neither of these family members was ever supportive of the life decisions she made. In childhood, her father was always very critical of her. Sometime ago, her brother picked up on this and became quick to find fault with her when they were together. For years, Suzy lived away from home. During that time, her panic attacks were few and far between. Several years ago, she returned to her hometown. Shortly after that, her panic attacks began to increase in number and intensity. When she had an attack, it was usually in the car with her father and brother.

As her father started questioning her decisions regarding her divorce, Suzy began to feel totally out of control. As a result, her unconscious mind stepped in and took over, not only to protect her, but to assist her in regaining control. As the adrenaline began to race through her body, the "flight-or-fight" sensation became very strong, and the physical manifestations of the attack intensified. It was at this point that immediate action had to be taken. Suzy had to get out of the car. Her panic attack also forced her father to stop chastising her. Suzy's unconscious mind had taken control of the situation in order to get her out of an uncontrollable environment. Once out of the car, away from her father, her heart rate slowly returned to normal while her breathing relaxed. As her body calmed down, she was no longer sweating, and her thinking process cleared.

Although Suzy's panic attack appeared to put her in an out-of-control state, in the long run it enabled her to regain control of the situation. What an incredibly creative defense mechanism!

— **Explore your own panic attacks to determine why they're currently a "necessary" part of your life.**

- Write out in detail what your last few panic attacks have looked like. Are there any similarities? Do specific situations, triggers, environmental factors, foods, animals, sexual activities, themes in movies, times of day, ndividuals, the physical appearance of certain persons—including sex or age, tone of voice, or other factors—

seem to be consistently present when you have a panic attack? Really make an effort to document the different aspects of your attacks.

• Try to observe yourself while you're having an attack. During a panic attack, imagine that there's a part of yourself in the distance, watching you as you go through this experience. Give this part of yourself physical form, and imagine this "you" watching you from a mountaintop, cloud, or corner of the room. After the attack, ask the image of yourself watching you, "Why did I have this attack? What is the panic attack protecting me from?" Listen carefully to what is said and then be sure to write down the answers on a sheet of paper.

Lifestyle Remedies for Panic Attacks

— **Safety, please.** Panic attacks are usually more prevalent when one is not feeling safe. Not feeling safe produces an "out-of-control" sense of being, and as we have learned, these attacks are tied to a feeling of loss of control. When we're unable to control our lives, we'll feel anxious. *Anxiety* is another word for *fear*, and at the base of a panic attack is the emotion, fear. By reducing your level of fear and increasing your sense of safety, panic attacks can be minimized.

Take out another piece of paper. List the people and places you encounter on a daily basis. After you've done so, ask yourself whether or not you feel safe when in these places or with these people. Put a star next to each person or place on your list that elicits a feeling of anxiety, fear, or lack of safety.

Next, think of ways in which you can limit your contact with the "starred" people, places, and things on this list. If you cannot limit contact, write out ways in which you can take care of yourself in these instances. What do you need to do to feel safer when confronted with these people, animals, items, situations, or activities? By understanding what triggers your panic, you can develop a plan of action to minimize your attacks.

— **Connect with others.** List all of your friends and relatives on a sheet of paper. Who on this list could you call for support if you found that you were experiencing the beginnings of a panic attack? When your breath begins to constrict, your heart is pounding, anxiety is permeating your thinking, or when you're overwhelmed with fear and tears, could you call them? If so, get ready to make use of your cell phone.

When you feel a panic attack overtaking you, immediately go to a safe place. If you're at work, head for the rest room, lunch area, or an outdoor area. As you make your way to a safe place, be sure to grab your cell phone. If panic hits at home, pick up a nurturing object (special blanket, pillow, stuffed animal, or whatever provides you with a sense of comfort) to cuddle with. Try to carry your list of phone numbers with you at all times—in a pocket, purse, wallet, schedule, or pocketbook. Once you're in a safe place, start dialing. It's extremely important for you to have several people on your list. If no one is home, talk to their answering machine. Express your anxiety and fear. Cry if you need to. As you continue to talk, your anxiety will begin to dissipate. Having people around who you can vent to often diffuses a panic attack.

After an attack, try to figure out what set it off, how it protected you, and in what way it interfered with your plans for that day. End your writing with an essay on what you've learned from this particular panic attack.

— **Inducing a panic attack.** In order to get around panic attacks, sometimes we must walk straight through them. This psychological consideration is useful if you're in therapy with a nurturing, supportive caregiver who can keep you in the here-and-now as you walk through this process. In my private practice, I will often induce a mild attack with individuals who suffer from panic attacks. I begin this process by asking the person to close their eyes and visualize in their mind, their concept of God, a Higher Power, angels, or guides. This provides a sense of safety during the experience. The client is then asked to visualize those triggers (animals, claustrophobia areas, being lost, work situations, people, sexual encounters, movies) that bring on an attack. With this, a controlled panic begins to build. During this time, I continually remind the person that they are safe, nobody is going to hurt them, they will not die, their feelings cannot destroy them, and that they can stop this process anytime they want to.

Once the anxiety has reached a high, I suggest they build a Plexiglas jail cell around the trigger item. They are then encouraged to really focus in on the person, place, or thing triggering the attack and ask, "Why am I so afraid of you?" If necessary, I suggest that they scream this question at the trigger. They're also encouraged to see themselves physically growing very big, stomping on the trigger, and demanding an answer. This particular empowering visualization can dilute anxiety and fear. After listening for an answer, it's then time to open the eyes and begin writing about the experience.

(**Note:** Do not attempt to take this step on your own. Having another person "witness" your experience as you move through this process is essential for your healing. Take the above step with your spiritual advisor, therapist, or health-care provider at your side. Such a person will be able to give you encouragement when you become frightened, and offer grounding if you feel you're getting lost in the panic. Here-and-now statements such as, "I am here," and hand-holding can be extremely reassuring. Asking for help takes a great deal of courage, but I know you'll be able to do it.)

Our emotions can greatly impact the intensity of panic attacks. As we've seen, we don't have to hand over our sense of safety and control to these attacks. By understanding what emotional triggers contribute to this painful state of being, we can begin to unravel the mystery behind this devastating condition. What we put into our physical bodies can also lead to panic attacks. It's now time to look at the nutritional and herbal remedies available for our healing.

Nutrition and Herbs to Assist in Reducing Panic Attacks

— **Avoid stress-inducing foods.** Caffeine stimulates the body and increases anxiety. It always fascinates me to talk with someone suffering from acute anxiety attacks as they sit with a caffeinated drink in hand. When I suggest that possibly the excessive amount of cola, coffee, or tea might be contributing to their panic attacks, they look at me dumbfounded.

If you suffer from panic attacks, stay away from anything that contains caffeine. That sweet brownie for dessert or the chocolate yogurt at lunch can contain large amounts of caffeine. Try sipping herbal teas or juices instead of caffeinated beverages. Also, many popular headache remedies found in drugstores contain massive amounts of caffeine. Start reading food labels, and become educated about what your favorite food products contain. A diet high in caffeine leaves little room for calming foods such as complex carbohydrates, and those rich in calcium and magnesium.

A doctor friend of mine was drinking quite a bit of coffee in the mornings. One day, after performing surgery for several hours, he started to have a panic attack and thought he was having a heart attack or stroke. Grabbing his nurse, he insisted she take his vitals. When he shared this dramatic tale with me, the first question I asked him was, "How much caffeine did you have that morning, and what did you have to eat?" My doctor friend had skipped breakfast and instead had slowly drunk several cups of strong black coffee.

— **Avoid the sugar buzz.** Ingesting pure, white, or brown processed sugar is like sticking your fingers into a light socket. Yes, you get zapped and then suffer dearly afterward. White sugar stresses an already stressed body and is completely void of nutrients. Pure, processed sugar quickly floods your cells and leaves you totally uninterested in foods that are good for you. Craving for sugar increases if you continue to make sugary snacks a daily habit.

If you have an overpowering desire for sugar products, get a hold of some **Chromium picolinate.** Taking 200 mcg per day of this nutrient not only reduces anxiety, but it will help with sugar cravings.

— **A diet high in whole, fresh, fibrous foods.** Complex, starchy carbohydrates have a calming effect on the body. One of my favorites is **spelt,** a wonderful grain making a huge come-back. At one time in history, spelt was more popular than wheat. Spelt is a very nutritious whole food, containing more protein than wheat. It's used to make bread products, crackers, pasta, and a variety of cereals. This product can be found in your local health food store and on the shelves of many grocery stores. If a panic attack is beginning to bud, grab a couple of slices of whole-grain spelt bread, find a quiet place, take a couple of deep breaths, close your eyes, and visualize pushing the panic away. Then open your eyes and enjoy the taste of spelt.

The diet should also be rich in fresh vegetables; soy products (such as tofu, soy nuts, and soy milk); yogurt; legumes; fresh fruits; nut butters; and if you're not a vegetarian, small amounts of very lean poultry, meats, and fish. Also, you might want to check with your health-care provider to see if you suffer from blood-sugar disorders such as hypoglycemia or diabetes. This can greatly contribute to anxiety. If you find that you *do* have a blood-sugar disorder, daily **spirulina tablets** can balance out this difficulty. Also, rather than eating three large meals a day, eat several small meals throughout the day. This, too, will assist your body in maintaining a balanced blood-sugar level. If blood sugar is where it's supposed to be, your chances of getting cranky or breaking out in a panic will diminish considerably.

— **Food allergies.** For the next two weeks, document everything you put into your body. During this same period, note any physical or mood changes that occur. **Allergies to wheat, eggs, dairy, strawberries, melon, bananas, nuts, chocolate, alcohol, and other food products can contribute to panic attacks.**

(**Note:** Many cold medications and nasal sprays can create a state of anxiety. Also, the herb **ephedra** should be avoided.)

— **We can supplement our diet to calm down.** Although many people find that their panic attacks lessen if they just change their diet, some individuals need an added boost of nutrients from supplements. Along with a good multivitamin, consisting of all 22 vitamins and 20 minerals, here are some other nutrients to consider:

Taking 2,100 mg of **calcium** and 900 mg of **magnesium** per day, divided into three doses, will have a soothing effect on the nervous system. **Vitamin B complex** is necessary for maintaining proper function of the nervous system. Take as directed on the label. Extra **Vitamin C** can have a positive, calming effect, and it helps relieve anxiety. Taking 6,000 mg per day, divided into three doses, will also assist your body in dealing with everyday stress. **L-glutamine** is a wonderful amino acid that has mild tranquilizing effects. The suggested dose is 500 mg with a large glass of water on an empty stomach, three times per day.

Finally, I cannot end this section without briefly discussing the hormone **melatonin.** As we begin that trek toward middle age, our natural production of melatonin begins to drop. Melatonin is not only a wonderful antioxidant, but it can induce sleep. Although melatonin levels rise naturally in the body as the darkness of night approaches, some individuals can benefit greatly by supplementing with this hormone. If you suffer from restless sleep patterns, try taking 2 mg of melatonin an hour or two before bedtime. If this dose does not seem to promote a restful sleep, you can raise the dose by 1 mg per night until you determine what amount works for you. It's suggested that doses above 10 mg not be used. If you are prone to panic attacks, you may find that melatonin is also useful in treating the sleep disturbances that can contribute to these attacks.

(**Note:** Do not use this supplement if you have an autoimmune disease or disorder, and do not use melatonin with children.)

I strongly suspect that these small changes in your nutritional well-being will begin decreasing the number and intensity of your panic attacks. If the physical body is nurtured, properly fed, and well cared for, the mind can relax. Speaking of relaxing, there are numerous herbal remedies that are very effective for panic attacks.

— For mild relief of anxiety, try the herb **hyssop.** This fragrant plant was used by the Hebrews and Greeks for religious purification. Use it as a tea, three times a day.

(**Note:** Do not use hyssop if you suffer from epilepsy or a seizure disorder. Do not take the essential oil of this herb internally.)

— Have you ever watched a cat play with a **catnip** plant or toy? This is a wonderfully safe herb that brings felines of all ages hours of pure, purring kitty cat pleasure. In centuries gone by, when life became overwhelming, the dried leaves of the plant were smoked to induce a calm, relaxed state of mind in people. Keep this herb on hand for those moments when a panic attack is building. Try to carry the tea bag in your purse or wallet.

— **Vervain** has long been used to relieve anxiety and tension. A sacred herb of the Druids, it was once used regularly to ward off bad luck. Vervain is a wonderful restorative herb for the nervous system. Also, it's a useful remedy for tension headaches. In tincture form, this herb can also be carried in the pocket or purse. Take it in a glycerin tincture form three times a day, as directed on the label. (**Note:** If you take more than the suggested dose, you could experience nausea and vomiting.)

— **Skullcap** is a well-known nerveine. If the above herbs do not relieve your panic attack symptoms, it's suggested that you try skullcap. This particular herb has been around for centuries and was first documented in 1576 by L'Obel, personal botanist to King James I. Skullcap can be found in tea bag form in any health food store. Drink it three times a day. If your panic attacks are particularly intense, switch from the tea to capsules.

(**Note:** If you use more than the recommended dosages of this herb, sleepiness can occur. Also, never use skullcap if you're taking traditional mood-altering medications such as tranquilizers, antidepressants, or painkillers.)

With panic attacks, traditional drug therapies treat only a small part of the individual. The medications used often leave one with a kind of "blunted" feeling. Don't you deserve to be totally present for your life? There are joyful experiences to be had, and lessons to be learned for all of us. In my opinion, strong pharmaceutical medications should be used only when all other options have been exhausted. Doesn't it make sense to explore a more holistic approach first?

Suzy decided to see a physician who understood that treating the total person was the key to healing. Slowly, this doctor detoxed her off of all the anti-anxiety medication she was taking. With his help, she was then able to seek out a number of alternative solutions to her situation.

The following Thanksgiving, things were a lot different. "Yes," she said to her doctor, "I'm having Thanksgiving at my house, on my turf. And I've invited a lot of my friends. My buddies will balance out the dysfunction of my family."

Intrigued, her doctor asked, "How?"

Suzy laughed and then replied, "None of my family would dare say one inappropriate or critical thing to me in front of my friends. Heavens, no! Trust me, Doc. They will all be on their best behavior. Yes, my panic attacks served me well, but thankfully I no longer need them to rescue me from my family."

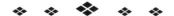

*C*hapter nine

SLEEP PROBLEMS AND THE FEAR OF GIVING UP CONTROL

Pat was fast asleep under a stack of colorful afghans and quilts. Two young orange-colored tabby cats snored softly near the head of her bed. Without warning, Pat's large golden retriever, Moose, jumped up on top of all of them. Both cats, rudely awakened, began to hiss and spit, forcing Pat to leave the delightful realm of dreamland. Sitting up, she pushed all of her animals off her bed. Turning to her right, she noticed that her husband, Paul, was nowhere to be seen. As she slid her feet into her pink bunny slippers, a recent Christmas present from Paul, she looked up at the clock hanging on the wall. Ding. Ding. Ding. *It's 3 o'clock in the morning. Where on earth could he be?* Pat wondered.

As she made her way down the stairs of her cozy two-story home, Pat saw the white light of the TV streaming toward her from the family room. "Not again," she sighed. Walking into the lighted room, she heard the distinct musical theme from a rerun of the television program *The Addams Family*. Turning to the couch, Pat saw her husband's 6'4" frame stretched out. On the television, Morticia, looking as ghoulish as ever, whirled a dagger toward her husband, Gomez. Pat sat down next to her husband, gently patted his leg, and asked, "Can't sleep again?"

If you're having difficulty sleeping, you're not alone. The National Commission on Sleep Disorders Research (NCSDR) has determined that approximately 40 million of us suffer from some type of sleep difficulty. Sleep problems can include **insomnia**, or difficulty falling asleep and staying in a sleep state; **restless leg syndrome**, or numbing of the legs and feet; and **sleep apnea**, where breathing actually stops for a period of seconds. It's normal to periodically suffer from insomnia. As we lay our heads down to sleep at night, now and then the stress of life can catch us all off-guard. When this happens, a sound sleep occurs the following night, restoring us to a restful state the next morning. Unlike common bouts of periodic insomnia, chronic insomnia can be persistent, plaguing us night after night, dramatically affecting our physical and psychological state.

The Psychology of Sleep Difficulties

In search of solutions to lack of sleep, many of us have made our way to traditional health-care providers. Most traditional caregivers are all too quick to pull out the prescription pad and then write out orders for potentially addictive, dangerous tranquilizers, antidepressants, and other sleep-inducing medications. Not only are most of these strong drugs habit-forming, but they can also have numerous other side effects, including morning confusion, weakness, dizziness, depression, stress on the liver, blood abnormalities, and decreased sex drive. Before popping a pill, let's look at the psychology behind sleep problems.

— Many sleep difficulties, especially those that are long-standing, have their **origins in childhood**. If one has had problems sleeping as a child, adolescence, or young adulthood, this difficulty can carry on into adulthood. When this is the case, the question to ask is, "Why do I have such a fear of giving up control and drifting off to sleep?" The following visualization can quickly resolve this issue.

While sitting in a comfortable room with no distractions, close your eyes and visualize walking into a log cabin in the mountains. It's nighttime, and the cabin is full of children and adults. All of these people are actually "you" at different ages. Some are sleeping, while others are wide awake. Notice who is awake, and then ask, "Why are you not sleeping like the others?" When you receive an answer, open your eyes and write it down on a piece of paper. It's possible that an unresolved life event or issue is in need of your attention and resolution. Sleep difficulties often have their origins in our past.

— Sleep difficulties can also be the result of **stressful here-and-now problems**. Once your head hits the pillow, divorce, continual job stress, an unresolved argument with a loved one, financial worries, or the fear of recurring nightmares can be just a few of the reasons why "letting go" feels impossible. The unresolved emotions related to current-day problems can keep us up night after night. The following visualization is useful for this situation.

Sit in a comfortable place, with your eyes closed. Visualize yourself sitting across from an image of yourself. Ask this other vision of you, "What's bothering you?" Listen very carefully. After hearing what is said, imagine telling this person that you will help them work through these concerns, and then thank them for sharing. Open your eyes, and write down all of your unresolved difficulties.

— When you find that you've been lying in bed for 30 minutes and are still wide awake, get out of bed. **Lying in bed actually worsens the situation.** Instead of suffering, go to another room and write a letter to God, your Higher Power, spiritual guides, the universe, angels, or your higher self about your frustration related to not being able to sleep. Write until you feel exhausted, and then return to bed.

After discovering those life issues that are in need of your attention, it's important to write out a plan of action. This plan should include methods for working out problems. If the solutions seem elusive, discuss these concerns with a therapist, spiritual advisor, rabbi, minister, close friend, or support group.

Addressing the psychological issues behind sleep disturbances will not resolve insomnia if certain lifestyle behaviors continue. How we live our lives during the day will greatly impact whether or not we will get to enjoy ZZZ-ing at night. To promote a nightly journey into dreamland, here are some simple lifestyle suggestions.

Lifestyle Remedies for Sleep Problems

— **Cut down on caffeine.** Colas, teas, coffee, and chocolate contain large amounts of this stimulating drug. This chemical can stay in the body for up to ten hours. If you must drink caffeine, try to abstain from it after lunch. Many people are very addicted to caffeine and find the thought of giving up their afternoon tea or coffee break overwhelming. If this is the case, try drinking coffee, teas, or colas that have only a 50 percent caffeine content.

Also, beware of that luscious-looking piece of chocolate cake just before bed. One piece of chocolate cake can contain as much as 20–30 mg of caffeine. Also, a number of over-the-counter medications contain this stimulant. For years, my grandfather took a certain headache remedy every night and then often wondered why he had such a difficult time getting to sleep. This particular headache medication contained 130 mg of caffeine. Two of these little pills contained more caffeine than a cup of espresso.

— Watch out for **cigarettes** and **alcohol.** Many people believe that a glass of wine or a brandy before bedtime will ensure a restful night's sleep. Wrong. Once the effects of the alcohol have worn off, the rebound effect can leave one "owl-eyed" and awake in the middle of the night. Alcohol use interferes with the deep-sleep cycle, necessary for restoring our physical and emotional well-being.

Cigarettes are also stimulating to the nervous system. Toking and puffing before "hitting the hay" can overstimulate the nervous system. If you smoke, try to abstain from smoking before bedtime.

— **Exercise, exercise!** No, you don't have to become an Olympic athlete, but a morning exercise routine can encourage a good night's sleep. Walking, bicycle riding, light weight lifting, swimming, hiking, folk dancing, window-washing, or any other physical activity is encouraged.

(**Note:** Exercising two to four hours before bed can make falling asleep difficult. Active physical activity encourages the release of adrenaline, a natural stimulant found in the body. When this stimulating chemical is flowing through our veins, sleep can be hours away.)

— **Excessive mental and emotional stress** can interfere with a good night's sleep. An upsetting phone call, an argument with a loved one, or a violent television program are just a few of the stresses that can ward off nighttime drowsiness. Never stay in bed ruminating over such concerns. Get up and write about it. After doing so, make a pact with yourself to address these strong emotions *tomorrow*. Imagine putting all of these concerns in a room and closing the door. Tell yourself that these issues will have your full attention the next day, after you've had a good night's sleep.

— **A warm bath or shower** can be very soothing for the mind and relaxing for tense muscles. Warm water actually encourages the blood vessels in the body to dilate, promoting an overall sleepy sensation. Taking a warm 30-minute soak in a scented bath several hours before bedtime is highly recommended. Lavender, one of the herbs taken to the New World by the Pilgrims in 1620, can encourage a delightful sleep. To relieve stress and tension, add five drops of lavender essential oil to a warm bath. The essential oil of this herb can also be applied to a handkerchief and then inserted between a bed pillow and the pillowcase. The scent is very calming. **Chamomile** and **geranium** essential oils can also be used in the bath.

Before stepping into scented bathwater, turn on some soothing music—a tune with a slow, methodical rhythm. The rhythm of such music often lowers blood pressure, slows down the heartbeat, and encourages a restful state of mind.

Several hours before bedtime, reduce the glare of any intense light. Bright light is very stimulating. Allowing "wind-down" time before going to bed with a scented bath, peaceful music, and soft lights gives the body and mind time to slow down.

— **Avoid greasy, heavy foods before bedtime.** A high-fat meal several hours before bed will not only jump-start the metabolism, leaving you in a restless state, but will also increase the heart rate and wreak havoc on the gastrointestinal system. Even if you do fall into a light sleep, greasy, heavy foods have a tendency to remind us of their presence in the middle of the night with gas, heartburn, and an upset tummy.

— **Create a safe bedtime environment.** I disagree with the experts who say it's not acceptable to fall asleep in front of the television. For some people, the TV distracts them from their worries, allowing sleep to creep in. One man told me, "Nothing puts me to sleep faster than a boring sitcom." The moral of this story is, "If it works, use it." For some people, a night-light can help create a sense of safety. With others, a few extra pillows will do the trick. Inviting pets to sleep in the room can be reassuring. A comforter with special meaning, or a family afghan, also offers security. Creating a safe sleeping environment can make the process of "letting go" a bit easier.

— **Meditation.** By learning to clear the mind with meditation, one can enter a peaceful sleep. With practice, dropping off to sleep occurs with ease. For the person who needs a bit of direction, there are numerous guided visual meditations available on tape at most bookstores. Along with these, there are tapes that provide instruction on self-hypnosis, which can also be a useful sleep aid.

— **Try to avoid napping.** Napping during the day will only make falling asleep at night more difficult. If drowsiness hits in the middle of the day, take a walk around the office or the neighborhood. Breathe deeply, filling the lungs with oxygen. Then have a large glass of iced spearmint herbal tea.

Nutritional and Herbal Support for a Good Night's Sleep

When individuals in our society go to a traditional health-care provider with a complaint about sleep problems, they are rarely told to investigate their diet. However, what we put into our body dramatically affects our sleep patterns. Let's take a look at just how nutrition impacts our ability to get the seven to eight hours of nighttime ZZZs we need for optimal health.

— Be sure to review the "Healthy Body, Well Mind" diet plan in Appendix I to see what constitutes a well-balanced daily diet.

— Caffeine isn't the only food product that can keep us awake, counting those sheep. Some foods contain chemicals that increase the release of **norepinephine, a brain stimulant**. The chemical **tyramine**, found in ham, cheese, sausage, chocolate, and even wine, increases the release of this stimulant. Individuals sensitive to norepinephine need to avoid these foods before bedtime. In order to determine whether you're sensitive to this chemical, remove the above foods, along with sauerkraut, eggplant, potatoes, sugar, tomatoes, and spinach from your evening meal for two weeks.

— Being **overweight** can also impact sleep, especially if this condition affects breathing. People who are overweight are at risk for **sleep apnea**. Although it is more common among middle-aged men, it can strike any seriously overweight person. With this disorder, the individual will snore. The snoring builds and gets louder, then suddenly, the person stops breathing and wakes up. This cycle can repeat itself over and over again throughout the night.

— Eat your bananas, which contain **tryptophan**. This amino acid increases the production of **serotonin,** a chemical that not only reduces stress, but also regulates sleep. If you don't like bananas, try having a few dates, figs, whole-grain crackers, soy milk, brown rice, or peanuts just before bed. Dairy products contain tryptophan. Grandmother's old remedy of a cup of heated milk, doused with a touch of vanilla flavoring and then topped off with just a tad of nutmeg, can induce a good night's sleep.

Complex carbohydrates will also help tryptophan enter the brain. That's why a turkey or peanut butter sandwich will make you sleepy.

— Believe it or not, being deficient in certain vitamins or minerals can greatly impact nightly sleep. Be sure to consider the supplements suggestions in this book, and only increase the dosages of those discussed in this chapter.

— **Restless leg syndrome,** with the nightly jerking and cramping of leg muscles, can be miserable. This syndrome can often be remedied with an increase in **calcium** and **magnesium,** and these nutrients are recommended for any sleep difficulty. Because calcium regulates nerve impulses, it has a calming effect on the nervous system. Magnesium not only relaxes the muscles, but is also needed to balance calcium. Taking 750–1,000 mg of calcium and 200 mg of magnesium at lunchtime, and an hour or so before bedtime, will promote a good night's sleep.

(**Note:** If you have kidney disease or a history of kidney stones, calcium supplements are not recommended. Also, calcium supplements can interfere with calcium channel blockers, often prescribed for high blood pressure and heart conditions.)

— **B vitamins** are stress-reducing nutrients. B3 (or niacin) is essential for a healthy nervous system, while B5 (or pantothenic acid) improves the body's ability to handle stress. Deficiencies in the Bs can produce insomnia. Increasing the daily intake of **Vitamin B complex** will promote relaxation and sleep at night. Take as directed on the label.

(**Note:** Vitamin B3 or niacin should be used with caution by those suffering from liver disease, glaucoma, diabetes, gout, or peptic ulcers. Doses over 500 mg should be avoided.)

— **Melatonin.** This supplement can be found in most drug and herbal stores. Taken in small doses, it appears to be a safe remedy for insomnia. Melatonin is actually a hormone that is produced naturally by the brain. For people over 65, Melatonin production is often depressed, causing insomnia. Although recommended doses vary, it's suggested that one begin with the smallest dose of this supplement. Start with 1.5 mg one hour before bedtime. If this is not effective, increase the dose to 3–5 mg.

(**Note:** Never take this nutritional supplement during the daytime or when driving at night. Excessive nighttime doses will cause grogginess in the morning.)

Herbs have long been used to combat sleepless nights. Numerous herbal remedies can be found at many health food stores, drugstores, and even grocery stores. Before going any further, it must be understood that sleep-inducing herbs can be as powerful and as toxic as over-the-counter or prescribed sleep medications. With this in mind, the following herbal remedies should be used with care, and they should *never be taken* if you are using tranquilizers, antidepressants, muscle relaxers, or sleep or pain medications.

— **Passion flower** can be an effective sleep remedy. According to herbal lore, the flowers of this herb were thought to represent the crucifixion or "passion" of Jesus, with the white and bluish purple colors representing purity and heaven. For insomnia, up to two cups of tea can be taken in the evening.

(**Note:** Excessive doses can cause nausea.)

— **Skullcap,** an herb used extensively by the Cherokee Indians, is a nerveine, and it will calm the nervous system. This herb can be used in tea, capsule, or tincture form an hour before retiring for the night. Use as directed on the label. Skullcap can also be used in combination with **chamomile**, a plant dedicated in ancient Egypt to the sun god Ra; and **hops**, an herb well known to the beer-drinking crowd. Chamomile tea is an extremely safe sleep remedy, and it has a long history of being used for sleeplessness in children. **Hops** can slow down a racing mind. A tea or tincture of the three above herbs is extremely useful for insomnia. (**Note:** If you are allergic to ragweed, avoid chamomile.)

— **Kava kava.** The root of this plant continues to be chewed and fermented with saliva by some islander groups in the South Pacific. Fortunately, we don't have to resort to the "chew and spit" method to experience the calming effects of this herb. For sleeplessness, use kava kava in tea, tincture, or capsule form. Take as directed on the label an hour before bedtime.

(**Note:** If taken in excess, this herb can produce a narcotic effect. Do not exceed the suggested dose.)

When sleep difficulties are treated with a holistic approach, the quality of your nighttime dreaming hours will be much improved.

Paul finally overcame years of insomnia by implementing the above program. Rarely did he miss a night's sleep.

It was Saturday afternoon, and Pat had just finished her grocery shopping. She was tired and needed help taking in the shopping bags. *Where is my darling husband?* she wondered. Pat found Paul sitting on the couch with Moose, the dog. The theme from *The Addams Family* was playing. This time Gomez was pitching daggers at Morticia. Shaking her head, Pat said, "Those two need some serious marriage counseling. Why are you watching this?"

Smiling, Paul responded, "Well, I can't watch it at night anymore, because now I'm sleeping!"

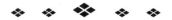

PART IV

*R*evitalizing
Reactive Kids

❧ ❧ ❧ ❧

Chapter ten

ATTENTION DEFICIT DISORDER: ALTERNATIVES TO RITALIN

It had been a very long day, and I was bone-tired. I had been booked back-to-back with client sessions, and, courtesy of my five-year-old, I was suffering from a head cold. As I sneezed into a handkerchief scented with the essential oils eucalyptus and peppermint, I thought to myself, *Two more hours and then a hot bath.* In the office across from mine, my husband, Michael, a child psychologist, was working with the parent of a very hyperactive boy.

Blowing my nose once more, I heard someone running at full speed up the stairs. Small footsteps then made their way down the staircase, soon returning back up. After grabbing another tissue, I stuck my head out of my office door and was suddenly confronted with a cute, cherub-faced little boy. Realizing this was the son of Michael's client, I asked, "Sweetie, would you please go into the playroom downstairs? Your mother will be out in a minute."

With an angelic smile, the little boy answered, "Okay," and then jumped to the bottom of the steps.

Returning to my office, I was about to take a sip of hot, vitamin-rich rose hip herbal tea when I heard *tromp, tromp, tromp* up the stairs, quickly followed by *clump, clump, clump* down the steps. Looking out of my office again, I watched my poor cat make a mad dash for the bottom of the stairs. Cat hair flew as she scrambled into the playroom to escape the clutches of the little boy. Following the two of them, I found the child flat on his stomach, with one arm reaching under an old, overstuffed chair. Although my furry friend had sought appropriate refuge from her pursuer, the angel-faced boy now had *me* to deal with.

The medical community believes that the stimulant Ritalin and other related medications effectively calm down ADHD (attention deficit hyperactive disorder) in children. Medical caregivers often push this particular mode of drug therapy on parents with problem youngsters. Michael works with many children who have been diagnosed with ADHD, and he is not supportive of stimulant drug therapy. In search of alternatives, parents often bring their children to him.

Within the last several years, there has been a dramatic increase in the use of Ritalin with school-aged children. One expert estimates that Ritalin use is up 700 percent compared to just five years ago. Why is it that suddenly so many children are being labeled with this disorder? The answer is simple. With overcrowded schools, teachers consistently find themselves with too many children to manage. When a child exhibits just a few of the many so-called symptoms of this diagnosis, educators quickly refer parents to a doctor for a prescription of the powerful medication Ritalin. Do we really need to be giving our children a medication that is also used to speed up the geriatric set?

The Psychology of ADHD

The "take a pill" mentality of traditional medicine has now made its way to the youngest members of our society. Because parents and caregivers want to do what's best for their kids, they're often too quick to listen to the uneducated suggestions of well-meaning teachers, educators, school counselors, psychologists, and medical professionals who insist that Ritalin is an absolute necessity. The symptoms on the current list for this diagnosis are varied and numerous. With such guidelines, I will venture to say that, periodically, the behavior of most children would appear to be symptomatic of ADHD. Ritalin may temporarily relieve some of these symptoms, but it's rarely the solution. Ritalin does not address the "whole person." Before prescribing a drug for ADHD, psychological issues, lifestyle, and nutrition must be explored.

— **Children are mirrors.** When we as adults are mad, glad, sad, afraid, or anxious, we're usually able to identify these emotions and do something about them. For the mind of a developing child, it's a different story altogether. Strong emotions can be difficult, if not impossible, for kids to sort out. Acting-out behavior is oftentimes a response to overwhelming emotions. These acting-out behaviors can include an inability to stay focused, excessive nervous tension, rage attacks, fighting in school, numerous emotional meltdowns with tears or lashing out, sleep difficulties, food disorders, excessive nail biting, bed-wetting, and difficulty staying on track at school or home.

In addition, children will often act out those emotions that their caregivers aren't addressing. Kids are like little feeling barometers. Although they may not understand adult or family difficulties, they can always sense when there are problems in a family system. Because children do not possess the maturity to sort out the emotions they see, or feel their parents experiencing, they will act-out with a variety of behaviors.

If you are the parent of a child who has been diagnosed with ADHD, make a list of all of the unresolved problems in your family. After you have done so, write down how you're handling these issues. When you're having difficulty with certain living problems, you can bet that your child will respond. If you feel that you can't work out your issues on your own, meet with a therapist or spiritual advisor who understands family system theory.

— **Consistent parenting.** Nothing sets a child off quicker than inconsistent parenting. Children need consistent structure. Even though they fight for control, deep inside they crave guidance. When we as caretakers are too strict or relaxed with discipline, this greatly impacts our children. Consistency provides kids with a strong sense of security. Knowing that someone much bigger than they are is in control provides young people with a feeling of safety. Often parents of ADHD-diagnosed youngsters will create wonderful guidelines and boundaries for their children, but then they won't stick with them. When children then act-out, these same parents may retaliate with incredible strictness to regain control of the situation. Such seesaw parenting can create immense emotional confusion and difficulty for kids. "I just don't know what I'm supposed to do," is a common complaint from many ADHD-diagnosed children.

As the parent of a child diagnosed with ADHD, it's also very important for you to really look at where your understanding of parenting came from. Sit down and make a list of all the parenting techniques your parents used with you. Take some time to reflect on how you were parented, and how you feel about the discipline you received. Did your parents listen to you? Could you tell them anything? How did they talk to each other? Did they express all of their emotions appropriately? Are you able to process your feelings in a healthy manner today?

Were your parents too tough on you or not strict enough? After you've completed this list, examine how your upbringing might be influencing your ability to parent your own children. If you discover you need help with parenting, contact a qualified child therapist or educator.

— **School days.** Recently, a client shared with me that her five-year-old son had received from his teacher a referral for evaluation for ADHD and Ritalin. The client, a bright, articulate, professional woman, had recently divorced her alcoholic husband. For months she had been working on establishing consistency in the home, for both herself and her young son. In spite of this, the father's drinking continued to greatly distress the young child. Aside from having a father plagued with alcoholism, the kindergartner had scored off the charts when he went through a battery of intelligence testing. As I visited with this client, she reported that her son was bored in school and felt he wasn't being challenged enough. Isn't it interesting that the school would immediately suggest that this child needed Ritalin before investigating his intelligence level or the emotional upset of his parents' recent divorce and the father's alcoholism? Thankfully, the child's mother was against using Ritalin. Alternative solutions were eventually implemented to increase her son's interest in school. In addition, psychological support assisted the boy in processing some of his feelings about his father's drinking.

Some children are visual learners, while others learn by listening. Of course we can't forget those children who are "hands-on" experiential learners. Sadly, in a traditional classroom setting, learning differences are not regularly taken into account. Most schools try to force students to master all tasks in the same manner. If a particular child isn't absorbing information like the others, this is often seen as a problem. When a child is having difficulty learning in the traditional way, such a youngster may appear unfocused, distracted, and disinterested in the material being presented. If there are difficult emotional issues confronting a child outside of the school environment, this, too, is a setup for acting-out behavior in the classroom. Will Ritalin solve the problem? Not in the long run.

For years I worked as a school psychologist and utilized numerous tests to determine which avenues of learning worked best for different kids. If the school psychologist in your district is unable to provide your child with such testing, visit a child psychologist or specialist who understands such matters. Once your child's abilities have been measured, talk with the school counselor about putting together a program of learning that will make school more interesting for your child.

— **Grief, trauma, and loss.** One out of every five children in this country experiences traumatic abuse. The symptoms of trauma can have ADHD characteristics. As a child, there was a great deal of emotional, physical, and sexual abuse in my family system. My sister Lila was diagnosed as hyperactive and put on Ritalin when she was very young. No one ever investigated the alcoholism or abuse in the family. The thought was, "Lila is just hyperactive. Put her on Ritalin and the problem will be solved." Tragically, Ritalin only masked the real issues my sister was grappling with.

If not properly addressed, traumas such as the death of a parent, grandparent, sibling, close friend, or pet; divorce; or a move to a different town or school can produce in a child reactions similar to ADHD symptoms. Assisting children in understanding their emotions will dramatically reduce acting-out behavior.

Lifestyle Remedies for ADHD Kids

Life can be very hectic. Between parents' work schedules and children's various activities, the modern-day family appears to be constantly on the go. The stress of such a lifestyle can begin to take its toll on everyone. As mentioned earlier, children tend to act-out their stress. If a child is very sensitive, the "go-go" American lifestyle can create behavioral problems.

— **Grounding in the home.** The home represents security and safety. When the world at large feels chaotic and frightening, children look to the familiarity of home to find order and relief. If their home life is unpredictable and disorganized, children can respond with numerous behavior problems. A disorganized environment will breed difficulties in focusing, tracking, and task completion for children. Here are a few guidelines to consider for making home life routine and consistent.

— **Minimizing changes.** A daily routine provides structure. Structure perpetuates a sense of security and safety. A feeling of security enables children to focus. The bedroom of ADHD children needs to be somewhat organized. Clothes should be in one place, with toys in another. Having a regular cleanup time encourages children to organize their environment. Parents should assist in this process, but not take over. The bedroom does not need to be perfectly maintained, just a bit orderly.

Breakfast, lunch, and dinner need to take place at the same time and place every day. If the family decides to have dinner out, it's strongly suggested that a parent sit next to the child. As a parent, you also provide transitional security. Your consistent presence makes change more bearable for your child. Yes, you are a security blanket.

Self-care activities such as brushing teeth and bathing need to take place with regularity. Also mapped out into a daily routine should be wake-up time, bedmaking, dressing, toothbrushing and bathing, breakfast, cartoons, departure for school, lunch, snacking, homework, chores, reading, and going to bed. This will provide a wonderful structure for your child. It will mean more work for you, but in the long run this will reduce your child's anxiety level and improve behavior.

Gather together colored paper, markers, and scissors. With your child, put together a colorful daily schedule. Map out your child's activities, hour by hour, day by day. Include home, school, and extracurricular activities. Try to create two of these schedules. Put one in your child's room and another in the kitchen. When your child comes to you feeling overwhelmed and unable to focus, walk her or him to the schedule to point out what should be happening at that time.

Finally, it's important to remember that you must always anticipate changes and prepare your child for them several days in advance. If there's going to be a change in routine, take time to discuss this with your child. One discussion is not enough. Several days of discussion will give your child time to emotionally adjust to the upcoming change in routine. When change *does* take place, understand that short-term behavior problems can arise and are normal.

— **Maintaining consistency in school.** As with the home environment, there must be consistency at school. Your child needs to have a teacher who is gentle but structured. If the teacher is reactive, emotional, and disorganized, your child will act-out this stress. Young kids love having a schedule at school. This gives them a sense of control. "First we read books, then we paint, and before lunch we do math." A grounded teacher produces grounded kids.

If your child is having difficulty focusing at school, try to determine what the root problem is. When school material is not challenging enough, bright kids often become bored. Boredom can lead to disruptive behavior. If the lessons are too advanced, this can be another setup for acting-out problems.

— **Balancing discipline and building self-esteem.** Healthy discipline sets boundaries with children. Healthy boundaries provide structure. Structure gives children security. Although children need boundaries and discipline, many parents are fearful of disciplining their own children. Setting boundaries in the family prepares children for life in adulthood. Saying no and not setting limits with children does a great deal of damage.

Establishing boundaries within the home is very simple, but it *does* take work. When children are acting-out, they need a warning, such as: "If you continue with this behavior, there will be a consequence." Wait several minutes, and then, if necessary, give one final caution: "This is your last warning. If the behavior continues, there will be a consequence. You have one minute." If the behavior still continues, you must then immediately institute a consequence and stick to it.

For small children, consequences must be brief and presented without delay. One minute for each year (in age) of time-out from cartoons, a favorite toy, or other play activity is appropriate. For older kids, consequences need to be a bit tougher. If eight-year-old Tim's current favorite toy is his bike, his consequence could be the loss of riding this bike for one to three days. After a time-out period, clarify the reason for the consequence, and then follow this with, "What can we do differently next time?" Be sure to praise appropriate responses.

Finally, always intervene before inappropriate behavior escalates. If you wait too long, your consequences will be meaningless. When giving your child instructions regarding behavior, they should be consistent and simple. Keep tasks to no more than three items at a time. For example, "Sally, I want you to hang up your dress, make your bed, and comb your hair." Have your child repeat these directions back to you. If this is too much at once, reduce the number of requests in your directions. And, yes, you *will* have to repeat yourself. After a task has been completed, be sure to acknowledge this with your child. "Wow! Your bed looks great." When a task has not been completed, redirect with positive statements such as, "Once your hair is combed, I'm looking forward to seeing how pretty you look," or "After you've made your bed, we can arrange all of your stuffed animals on it."

Solid boundary-setting with children builds healthy self-esteem. Teaching kids that there are consequences to inappropriate behavior encourages self-responsibility. Helping children express and discuss their emotions verbally can assist in keeping acting-out to a minimum. Now that we've taken care of the mind, let's see what we can do for the body.

Nutritional and Herbal Support for ADHD Kids

One mother of an ADHD child recently shared with me, "All she will eat is processed cheese, hot dogs, and potato chips." Upon hearing this, I thought, *Now there's fuel for ADHD behavior.* When treating this condition, diet is very important. If the diet is not addressed, very little will change.

— **Caffeine and sugar.** Caffeine and sugar do not *cause* ADHD, but they sure can contribute to it. Caffeine is a known stimulant. To give a child a sugary cola is an invitation for trouble. Caffeine causes restlessness and can increase irritability. Although it's not directly linked to ADHD, why add fuel to the fire?

Processed sugar (table sugar) contains zero nutritional value. Sugars are immediately absorbed into our system. When our cells are quickly flooded with sugars, we experience a burst of energy. Unfortunately, this burst of energy is short-lived, and blood-sugar levels then drop off suddenly, creating listlessness and fatigue. For children who have difficulty processing sugars or for those who may be hypoglycemic, low blood-sugar levels can encourage the body to release high amounts of adrenaline. This abrupt release of the "fight-or-flight" chemical attempts to compensate for low blood-sugar levels. This physical response can leave young children fidgety, agitated, and irritable. Since focusing is difficult for ADHD children, why add a lot of sugar to the problem? Cut down on the amount of sugar ingested. Stay away from sugary snacks, crackers, cereals, candies, pastries, and sodas. You won't be able to completely remove sugar from your child's diet, but every little bit helps.

— **Good food for a growing body.** Kids need nutritious foods to help them grow into healthy adults. Today's American-kid diet consists of fast foods laden with oil, food additives, and grease. Like adults, children need a diet rich in whole grains, vegetables, protein, and fruit. Healthy childhood nutrition isn't that difficult if you follow a few simple guidelines. Replace sugary, salty, fatty snacks with low-fat crackers, low-sugar nut butters, whole-grain breads, fruit, raw vegetables, and iced fruity herbal teas.

Encourage your children to be a part of the menu planning and cooking. This type of activity brings the family closer together, teaches children about nutrition and food preparation, and promotes self-esteem and responsibility. Finally, set an example. If you consume a junk-food diet, so will your children.

— **Those nasty food allergies and additives.** Most experts working with alternative treatments for ADHD agree that this condition can be dramatically influenced by food allergies and food additives. If your child craves a particular food, this could be an indication of a food allergy. Serious food cravings are a symptom of many food allergies. The quickest way to determine whether or not a food allergy is present is to remove from the diet those foods many ADHD children tend to react to. Dairy products; eggs; soy; wheat; foods containing the substance called salicylates (found in great concentration in apples, apple juice, grapes, grape juice, nuts, raisins); food preservatives such as BHT or BHA; artificial food colorings; and some food flavorings are just a few to begin with. Research by investigators such as Mary Ann Block has suggested that a large proportion of children suffering from ADHD symptoms are allergic to one or more of these foods.

Along with the above foods, remove all those with additives or artificial colorings from the diet for two to three weeks. Exchange wheat products for pure spelt, rice, or oat breads from the health food store. For dairy products, substitute rice milk, rice ice cream, and rice-based cheese products. Encourage the intake of hormone-free meats, poultry, and fish (these can be found at a kosher butcher shop or holistic grocery store), oats, oat products, and those fruits and vegetables not included in the above allergy list. After several weeks, see if there's a change in behavior. How is the child's concentration, focusing, school behavior, mood, and anxiety level?

Add one food per week from the allergy list back into the diet. During the week, if your child begins to have difficulty with ADHD symptoms; complains of headaches, stomachaches, rashes or itching; starts sneezing; develops a stopped-up or runny nose; or if you notice redness suddenly on the ears, you may suspect a food allergy.

— **Nutritional supplements and herbs.** Many children today are suffering from some type of nutritional deficiency. A good children's **multivitamin** may be necessary. Stay away from grocery-store chewables that are loaded with sugar. Go to the health food store and consult with a knowledgeable employee about low-sugar multivitamins for your child. Make sure your multivitamin contains all of the stress-reducing **B vitamins.**

Researchers have also discovered that many ADHD symptoms are the result of a deficiency in essential fatty acids (EFAs). A good source of EFA is found in **flaxseed oil**. One to two teaspoons per day, mixed in food, will provide your child with a healthy dose of EFAs.

If you have discovered that your child is lactose intolerant (allergic to dairy products), supplementing with **calcium** and **magnesium** is suggested. Research indicates that some ADHD kids are deficient in magnesium. Younger children can take 100 mg of magnesium and 400 mg of calcium before bedtime. Before hitting the sack, older children should take 200 mg of magnesium and 800 mg of calcium.

As we come to the end of this section on ADHD, let me mention some of the herbs that are beneficial for this condition. **Chamomile** has a long history as a useful children's herb. I've used chamomile with both my boys for restlessness and tummy aches. For younger children, steep one tea bag of chamomile tea in two boiling cups of water for 20 minutes. For older children, use one cup of boiling water per tea bag.

(**Note:** If your child responds to this tea with wheezing and a runny nose, try **catnip**. This herb is another very safe, age-old remedy for children. It supports the nervous system and has a calming effect. Catnip and Vitamin C-rich elderberry or lemon grass tea tastes yummy. Take one tea bag of catnip, along with one of **elderberry**. Place in a teapot and add four cups of boiling water. Then steep for 20 minutes. Use the above tea remedies as needed for ADHD symptoms.)

Hops in a glycerin tincture form is a wonderful remedy to keep in the purse or briefcase when traveling with your child. This safe herb has a gentle, calming effect on the nervous system. For young children, reduce the adult dose on the label to one-third. For older children, cut the dose to half of that of the adult dose.

Both Michael and I are beginning to see a connection between addiction to stimulant drugs in the teen years and use of stimulant pharmaceuticals such as Ritalin during the younger years. Time will tell if there truly is a correlation. In the meantime, before using powerful pharmaceuticals, doesn't it make sense to utilize holistic methods of healing for ADHD symptoms? If you need more information on alternative treatments for

ADHD, I recommend a wonderful book called *No More Ritalin* by Mary Ann Block (Kensington Books, New York, NY, 1996.)

My poor kitty cat stayed under the overstuffed chair in the playroom for the rest of the afternoon. After the cherub-faced boy's mother came down the stairs with Michael, I said, "Your child is sitting in my office, coloring. He got a bit wound up there. Do you think the cola and chocolate cookies in his backpack could be contributing to a bit of his difficulty?"

Sadly shaking her head yes, the pretty blonde answered, "Your husband said the same thing. I never thought his diet could be part of the problem." As she wiped a tear from her eye, she added, "Dr. Brandon shared a lot of information with me about alternatives to Ritalin. I can't tell you how relieved I am to hear this."

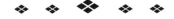

Chapter eleven

ADOLESCENT ACTING-OUT: WHAT'S IT ALL ABOUT?

James was a gangly-looking kid. With bright green hair and a nose ring, the young man sitting in my office might initially have been misjudged. On his forearm, I noticed an interesting tattoo. "When did you get that?" I asked.

The 16-year-old glanced at me with suspicion and replied, "Last summer."

Returning my gaze to the colorful art on his arm, I added, "It's good work," and then showed him the series of blue dolphins I had tattooed on my own leg.

Looking somewhat surprised, James let out a chuckle, shook his head, and leaned back on the couch. I had noticed that his tongue was pierced, so I continued this slow-moving conversation by asking, "Did that hurt?" With this question, I caught a look from him that said, "You must be dumber than dirt." Yes, this young man was angry, very angry, especially toward adults.

His father had told him that he had to come see me for therapy. James knew if he didn't keep our appointments, he would lose the keys to the family car. This was our second session together, and I was still "pulling teeth" for some sort of dialogue.

"Been to any good concerts lately?" I asked. Again, no response. In spite of his silence, I wasn't about to give up.

"My son had me pick up some alternative rock band's latest CD. I listened to it and loved the music. Next month, the two of us are going to see the group in concert."

With this, James stopped picking at the scab on his hand and replied, "What group?" *Finally*, I thought to myself. *An opening.*

As the sessions continued, James's hair color changed, he got a few more tattoos, and ended up having a lot to talk about. Two-thirds of each session rotated around rock bands, body piercing, and tattoo magazines. In addition, we managed to spend some of the time discussing his sister's death, the divorce of his parents, and the boredom he experienced at school. Yes, our talks became very productive.

Every week, angry, hostile, lonely, depressed, and often alienated adolescents cautiously walk through my office. Some of them have blue hair, while others are dressed in only the preppiest attire. A number of them are having difficulty at school, while others are making straight As. Many of these kids live with parents who have been married for decades, but a few report that Mom or Dad is on mate number five. In spite of these radical differences, all of these young adults have one thing in common: In one way or another, they're all "acting-out" certain emotions. And usually these feelings are emotions that they're incapable of dealing with.

The Psychology of Adolescent Acting-Out

— **What is acting-out behavior?** "I think he's smoking pot and drinking. What's next?" "She wants to pierce her ear again." "He freaked out because he got one B on his report card." "I found

out she's been having sex in her bedroom, right under my nose."
"His grades are awful. He doesn't seem to care." "She's cutting
herself with a razor blade. I don't know what to do." "He doesn't
respect the rules of this house; I'm beside myself." "She hit me. I
couldn't believe it. She hit me hard." "He was out all night again
and didn't tell me where he was going." "She gets good grades, is
very popular, and seems to be doing well, but I think she throws
up after every meal."

These are just a few of the concerns I've heard about kids
from parents over the years. In every situation, my first response
is, "Let's take a look at why your child is acting-out." If kids don't
know how to process certain feelings, they will act-out their emotions. Bad grades, self-destructiveness, addiction, sexual promis-
cuity, depression, isolation, and moodiness are often a cover for
fear, shame, anger, loneliness, confusion, alienation, grief, and
frustration.

Take out a piece of paper and ask yourself two questions:

• Can my adolescent child comfortably show emotion
  in a healthy manner?

• If my child doesn't know how to get angry, experience
  sadness, or express fear, how does she or he "act out"
  these emotions? Is it with rebellion, alcohol, drugs,
  bulimia, isolation, anorexia, extreme moodiness, compulsive eating, fighting, perfection, poor school behavior, a disrespectful attitude, or downright out-of-control
  actions?

After listing all of your child's acting-out behaviors, try to
determine what emotions are being expressed. Here's a hint:
James's green hair, tattoos, and piercings really upset his father.
He could never directly express his anger toward this parent, so
he acted this emotion out by doing those things to his body that

his father vehemently disapproved of. Was he consciously doing so? Maybe yes, but sometimes no.

If you have children who are acting-out their emotions, you may need to do two things:

- Look at how you express your feelings. Can you express all of your emotions in a healthy manner? If not, get some help to improve.
- Next, find a way to teach your children how to express emotion.

After realizing that I had difficulty handling my own anger, I learned how to do this in a healing, growth-producing fashion. I then passed these tools on to my children. Today, the anger emotion is accepted in our household if it's processed in an appropriate, nondestructive way.

— **Understanding adolescent separation.** My son Aaron is at an age where the process of separation and individualization is not only normal, but expected. Healthy adolescent separation occurs between the ages of 12 and 20. During this time, young adults are trying to figure out who they are, what they like, where they're going, and what they believe in. Children typically start this process by disagreeing with practically everything we as parents do or give credence to. Aaron not only thinks that I dress "weird," but he recently announced, "Classical music is just boring elevator music." Two years ago, before he began the developmental process of separation, he and I enjoyed listening to classical music together. Not anymore.

At this point in my son's development, it's his job not to like what I like. In order to find himself, Aaron must separate from me. In my son's mind, classical music represents "Mom." In order to separate from me, he has to openly state, "I don't like that type of music anymore." This is normal adolescent behavior, and it's often confused with acting-out.

Try to distinguish between acting-out behavior and separation. Many of today's kids attempt to separate from their parents by dyeing their hair a rainbow of colors and piercing holes in their bodies. They will do this because they know you don't like it. Always remember that hair grows back and pierced holes will close up. If necessary, tattoos can be removed with laser surgery. Underneath the black lipstick and blue fingernail polish resides the spirit of your lovable kid. If you focus too much of your attention on outside appearances, you will miss the many delightful changes that are taking place on the inside.

How we discipline our children can also directly impact acting-out behavior. This lifestyle issue is often neglected by the child psychologists and psychiatrists. Hopefully, you will take it to heart.

Lifestyle Remedies for the Acting-Out Adolescent

—**Overempowered versus disempowered kids.** In my opinion, the Baby Boomer generation has a difficult time setting appropriate limits with their children. Excessive material goods replace healthy boundaries, and consequences for unacceptable behavior are rarely enforced. Such parenting tends to produce overempowered kids who are often mouthy, disrespectful, demanding, and extremely self-centered. With adolescents like these, the life of the parents always rotates around them. A demanding young child eventually evolves into a very hard-to-please adolescent.

Controlling the behavior of a younger child is much easier than governing the conduct of an adolescent. If you have an overempowered adolescent, the road ahead will be difficult. As you begin your trudge down this path, you must begin by learning how to learn to say no to your adolescent. If you continue to give in when you should be setting limits, you will make matters more difficult. Assistance from parents' groups or a qualified health-care provider who understands adolescence may be necessary.

On the flip side of this coin is the disempowered child. On the outside, disempowered children usually appear to be the "good kids." Unfortunately they are often *too* good, and they have a tendency to grow into little "parents" or caretakers. By caretaking others, their own feelings of disempowerment or low self-worth are replaced by a false sense of empowerment. This behavior in adolescents leads to dysfunctional relationships in adulthood. Such adults look for people they can take care of, such as addicts, alcoholics, or low-motivated individuals. In adulthood, they end up sacrificing their own needs for the wants of others, and rarely take care of themselves.

Both disempowered and overempowered kids can often be very controlling. If you're being confronted with a child like this, you may need assistance in reclaiming your role as parent. Limiting this child's exposure to adult conversation, difficulties, and situations is a good place to start. The immature mind of an adolescent is incapable of processing adult information in a healthy way. Keep your adult world of relationship concerns, financial worries, ex-partner matters, and other mature family problems away from the ears of these kids.

Suggestions for Dealing with the Acting-Out Adolescent

— **Don't worry about the small stuff.** If your adolescent's room looks like a major disaster area, close the door. When your kids leave their belongings all over the house, don't go to war over it. Collect everything, put it in a laundry basket, and then put it in their room.

— **Keep the bedroom comforts to a minimum.** Too many parents overindulge their children with televisions, telephones, radios, CD players, computer games, and stereo systems. When adolescents have all of these technological goodies in their bedroom, they don't have to socialize with the rest of the family. Having a game room or central area for such mechanical contraptions keeps adolescents from isolating from the family.

— **Always remember that your child does not process emotion in the same way you do.** Never wait for your child to come to you. If you suspect there's a problem, there probably is. Your adolescent child does not have the problem-solving tools that you have. What you take for granted, such as the ability to work out a relationship dispute, will be elusive to your adolescent. Ask questions and don't settle for comments such as, "Okay," "Fine," "Nothing!" or "You wouldn't understand." If direct conversation and inquiry proves to be of little use, write your child a letter about your concerns. List in this note the concrete behaviors you're seeing. When your child *does* start to talk, really listen to what is being said. Listening is more important than giving direction. Be careful about talking "at" your kid. If you do this, you will be tuned out. Once your child is done talking, then offer several solutions. By the way, behaviors also provide big clues, so pay attention.

— **If you present a consequence for unacceptable behavior, stick with it.** My husband, as a child psychologist, has two rules for disciplining children. The first is, use leverage that will have a direct and profound impact. My son loves talking on the phone, which has provided his father and me with great leverage for consequences to inappropriate behavior—that is, suspending his phone privileges. (One client of mine refused to pay for driver's education until her daughter's behavior improved.)

Second, keep the length of the consequence within reason. If you ground your child for a month or take away all creature comforts for weeks, your consequence will lose its impact. Young people quickly adjust to change, and they tend to acclimate to intense disciplining measures. As Michael says so often, "Discipline should be to the point—short and sweet."

— **Communicate with all those who are involved with your child.** Don't hesitate to talk to teachers, coaches, family members, scout leaders, or other parents about your child's activities. What you don't know could hurt both you and your adolescent.

During adolescence, the body goes through numerous changes. Growth spurts and hormonal shifts can directly impact the behavior of a young adult. In addition, the body of a young person often bulks up right before a growth spurt. This extra body fat is normal, but many parents overreact and believe they have a "fat" kid on their hands. They then put the child on a diet. At this time of life, dieting is usually the last thing a kid needs. Understanding the physical transformations and nutritional requirements of adolescence does a great deal to alleviate misunderstanding, emotional outbursts, and unnecessary concerns.

Nutrition and Herbs to Assist in Reducing Acting-Out Behavior

— **Eating habits.** My son Aaron eats constantly. I often tell people I live at the grocery store. A 16-year-old boy needs 2,800 calories per day, while a girl of the same age requires 2,200 calories per day. Too many teens fall into the "media" trap and begin dieting in an attempt to look like models or celebrities. Other young people live on a fast-food diet consisting of burgers, hot dogs, greasy potato chips, french fries, and sugary sweets. Although fast-food drive-through restaurants are here to stay, we can still control what edibles enter the doorways of our homes.

To balance out society's current eating habits, I don't keep a lot of junk food in the house. Instead, I fill the refrigerator, pantry, and cupboards with items that are high in proteins, vitamins, and minerals; and low in sugars, fats, and salts. In my kitchen, one drawer is called the "snack drawer." When my boys open up this particular drawer, they know they can always find something interesting to snack on. Items such as low-fat and low-salt popcorn, nut butters, low-fat crackers, low-fat cheese spreads, and vitamin-rich breads or cereals low in sugar can be found in this "kid food" reservoir. In my refrigerator, fruit juices, fruity iced herbal teas, and bottled water replaces sugary sodas.

Many teens skip breakfast, and for this reason, it's useful to have little bags of vitamin-rich cereals or granola bars available in the morning. I often hand my sons such food items as they're walking out the door for school.

The nutritional level of school lunches is debatable. Just today I asked my oldest son, "What did you have for lunch?" His response was, "Pizza and fries." Because school lunches are often devoid of any nutritional value, wholesome afternoon snack foods are a necessity. Bowls of fresh fruit and cut-up carrot and celery sticks are wonderful grab foods for adolescents. Low-fat string cheeses in single-serving packets are another favorite around my house.

Dinner meals should be served early in the evening, and they need to be balanced with grains, starches, fresh seasonal vegetables, lean meat, dairy products, or vegetable proteins, and have as little sugar as possible. Don't forget evening snack foods. An hour or two after dinner, fortified cereals on top of low-fat ice cream or frozen fruit Popsicles usually hit the spot.

Foods rich in **calcium** are essential. Kids ages 8 to 18 need 1,200 mg of calcium per day. This mineral can be found in fortified breads, dark green leafy vegetables, and dairy products. If your teenager is allergic to milk products, there are many juices on the market that are enriched with calcium. Be sure to have reduced-fat milk, yogurt, cheeses, or calcium-rich fruit juices on hand at all times. Aaron has a large glass of orange juice every night before he goes to bed. If he finds that the orange juice container is empty, you can be assured that I hear about it.

— **Diet may not be enough.** In some situations, diet may not be enough. As teens age, they tend to spend more time away from home with friends and involved in other social activities. During this period, regulating a young person's diet can become impossible. A steady intake of pizza, candy bars, and other junk foods will eventually leave your adolescent deficient in necessary vitamins, minerals, and fiber. Bone formation alone demands adequate amounts of **Vitamin D, calcium, phosphorus,** and **protein.** These nutrients will not be found in a chocolate bar or doughnut. For the adolescent who's growing by leaps and bounds, nutritional supplementation is often necessary.

Unfortunately, making sure an adolescent takes nutritional supplements is easier said than done. In past years, I've cleared away my family's breakfast dishes only to find their supplements sitting, untouched. As a result, I've had to become both creative and devious. In health food stores, it's easy to find numerous vitamin and mineral supplements in liquid or spray form. Today, I spray a dose of multivitamins into my sons' orange juice. You can give supplements so that kids never even notice how Mom is lending them a nutritional helping hand. When the winter months roll around, colds and flus are common. During the cold season, I keep a Vitamin C spray handy at all times. The taste of this spray is pleasant, so all I have to say to my children is, "Open wide." If you decide to supplement your adolescent's diet with vitamins and minerals, make sure the doses are appropriate for your child's weight and age.

Over the last decade, more and more adolescents have been placed on strong medications. Antidepressants, stimulants, and a variety of other mood-altering prescription drugs are making their way into the veins of this country's youth. Does this solve acting-out behavior? In my opinion, no. What it does do is blunt emotion and possibly interfere with the developmental process. Like adults, young people can also benefit from medicinal herbs.

— **Popular herbs for children and adolescents.** If you were to walk into your local health food store, you would find one or two shelves devoted solely to herbal remedies for children. The popular medicinal herbs **chamomile, catnip,** and **oat straw** would be very visible. The scent of chamomile is similar to that of an apple, and this pleasant-tasting herb is quite safe for kids. The remedy is useful when anxiety strikes and emotions are on overload.

(**Note:** Do not use chamomile with adolescents who are allergic to ragweed or common grasses.)

Catnip, another child-friendly herbal remedy, has been used throughout the centuries to calm the nerves. This plant with the heart-shaped leaves is also useful for insomnia and stress. Speaking of stress, oats are not only for breakfast. **Oat straw** has antidepressant qualities and is a wonderful remedy for the moody or depressed adolescent.

At your local health food store, all three of these herbs can be found in glycerin tincture form. Add an age-appropriate dose of one of these herbal tinctures to a glass of juice or herbal tea, three times a day. Tinctures containing combinations of **chamomile, catnip,** and **oat straw** are also strongly suggested.

(**Note:** For adolescents 12 to 14 years of age, use half of the suggested dose on the label.)

Adolescence is such a rough time. The body is rapidly changing and independence is nearing. The shifting hormones can create an emotional meltdown in no time at all. The awkwardness of this age can be further complicated by the death of a loved one (even a pet), the divorce of parents, a change in schools, the rejection of a first love, and simply by the stress of modern living. Assisting young people in the transition from childhood to young adulthood takes patience and understanding, along with an ability to set boundaries and listen. If you find that you are having difficulty parenting an adolescent, don't hesitate to reach out for help from child therapists, church groups, other parents, and support groups such as Al-Anon or Co-dependents Anonymous. Finally, always remember that your guidance and support will help the adolescent in your life blossom into a loving, compassionate young man or woman.

James came into the kitchen, and I poured us each a cup of elderberry tea. As I reached for the honey, I heard James sigh. "You know, it only seems like yesterday that I was coming here," he said. As I spooned the sweet bee treat into our cups of tea, James continued. "How did you put up with me? Was I one of you more difficult cases?" With this, we both laughed.

"So, what are you doing with yourself these days?" I asked as I took a sip of the deep purple tea.

"I'm having the time of my life." he replied. "Right now I'm just coasting. Nothing serious. I live with a couple of other guys in a house down on the beach, and I'm working at a record store."

While stirring a bit more honey into my brew, I said, "That sounds like fun."

Princess, my spoiled kitty cat, came wandering into the kitchen, snubbed both of us, and headed for her food bowl in the other room. With a snicker, James said, "Well, I'm glad to see some things never change. She's as unfriendly as ever." Once again we both shared a chuckle.

After we had our tea, I walked James to the door. Before we

could make our way to the front porch, in walked my next client. Dressed in all-black, with pale face makeup, and black eyeliner and lipstick, one would have thought that this young girl was suffering from anemia. As she passed through the doorway, she gave James a quick "once-over" and then silently made her way to my upstairs office. Looking back at me, he quietly asked, "Was I that morose?"

With a smile, I gave him a final hug and said, "Yes, but I'd say you came through it rather nicely."

As he started to leave, he quickly turned around and said, "Thanks, Doc."

Waving good-bye, I said to myself, *Those two simple words make my job worth doing.*

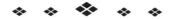

PART V

No Longer Hiding from Life

❧ ❧ ❧ ❧

Chapter twelve

SMOKING: A COVER FOR FEAR AND ANGER

The three women sitting at the table had been lunching together every month for more than five years. Joyce, an attractive 32-year-old redhead, was glaring at her friend Elizabeth, who was sitting across the table smoking a cigarette. "How can you sit there smoking that thing when your sister just had a lump removed from her breast?" Joyce asked incredulously. "Aren't you going to be 50 years old next month? You must have *some* concern about your health."

Stunned by this sudden verbal attack, Elizabeth, a feisty-looking blonde, quickly put her cigarette out and asked, "Why are you getting so upset? You smoke like a fiend. If this isn't the pot calling the kettle black, I don't know what is."

Shelly, a 46-year-old brunette, had just finished her lunch, and as she pushed her plate away, she looked angrily at Joyce and asked, "Have you told Elizabeth you're trying to quit smoking?" Quickly grabbing a breadstick, Joyce replied, "No, not yet."

Thanks to the surgeon general, most of us are aware that cigarette smoking is responsible for many of the illnesses plaguing our society today. If smokers continue to puff away on their favorite brand of cigarettes, cancer, cardiovascular disease, and a reduced life span are just a few of the possible consequences they can look forward to. This information has been around for decades, but in spite of this, many smokers still find it difficult to give up cigarettes. With less tolerance in society for smoking, cigarette smokers in need of a nicotine fix often find themselves relegated to dark parking garages; specified outdoor areas subject to rain, wind, heat, or snow; and tiny "smoking permitted" rooms.

Many smokers see the cigarette as their enemy and feel as though this little stick of tobacco is holding them hostage, forcing them to forever remain second-class citizens. As one woman told me, "I feel like a sinner every time I light up." A deep sense of shame often makes abstinence difficult and relapse common. Relapse continues because, like society in general, most smokers treat the cigarette itself as the problem. The thought is, "If I get rid of the cigarettes, my problem will be solved." If the smoker doesn't understand that every aspect of their physical, emotional, and spiritual being plays a role in maintaining a dependence on cigarettes, then the individual may end up being a smoker for life.

The Psychology of Smoking

— **Understanding this addiction.** At one time, smoking was considered a glamorous act. Scenes from Hollywood films—such as those with Humphrey Bogart and Ingrid Bergman in deep conversation in the classic film *Casablanca*—convinced many of us that smoking was the "hip" thing to do. In an attempt to "look cool" or "fit in," most smokers who picked up that first cigarette neglected to understand that the smoke filling their lungs contained an addictive property known as the drug *nicotine*.

Nicotine has been presented by the media and medical community as the "evil" that keeps the smoker "hooked." Although this is true, nicotine has also provided a number of individuals with a quick method for stabilizing strong, overwhelming feelings. Because nicotine represses the emotions anger and fear, the cigarette has been a lifesaver for many of us. As a result, it's imperative that the individual who's trying to quit smoking understand several basic facts about this dependence:

— **Cigarettes are not the enemy.** In fact, it's important to recognize that smoking has provided many gifts. Smokers should recognize that one of these gifts has been the repression of certain feelings. Before giving up cigarettes, new survival skills need to be developed to process these everyday emotions.

— **New survival skills can be learned.** Instead of picking up a cigarette when you're angry, you may need to punch a punching bag or stomp on an empty soda can. If fear strikes, a phone call to an understanding friend or several moments of meditation may be needed to calm the nerves.

— **Saying good-bye helps.** Finally, it's important to properly say good-bye to the cigarettes that for so long have served as friend, lover, reward, protector, and tension reliever. Grieving the loss of this longtime friend is very necessary. The following visualization can be very effective in assisting the smoker in letting go of cigarettes:

> *With closed eyes, visualize the cigarettes. Give them a personality, a life of their own. Tell them that you're grateful that they've been there for you during rough times. Visualize some of these hard times, and remember the calmness that a cigarette can bring about. Now visualize some of the negative consequences of smoking, such*

as illness, smelly clothes, stained teeth and fingers, and sitting on a concrete ledge in a parking lot because the physical body was in need of another dose of nicotine. Now visualize telling the cigarettes that it's for these reasons that you must let them go.

After this visualization, a "letting-go" ceremony may be necessary. Bury a pack of cigarettes in the backyard. Smash a favorite ashtray, or slowly tear up a pack of cigarettes.

Lifestyle Remedies to Assist the New Nonsmoker

Once an individual decides to quit smoking, a number of lifestyle changes must take place. Understanding the psychology behind cigarette addiction is useless if behavioral changes do not follow. Putting down the cigarettes is just the beginning of this process. The following lifestyle changes will support new nonsmokers in their efforts to remain smoke free:

— **Avoid secondhand smoke and environments where smoking is permitted.** Such environments can trigger a desire to smoke in the early days of abstinence.

— **For the first week of abstinence, take a daily steam sauna.** Check at local gyms and health clubs for the availability of such facilities. If a steam room is unavailable, sit on a chair in a shower stall with the water running as hot as possible. Place a towel over the top of the stall to trap the steam. The essential oils **eucalyptus** or **spearmint** are wonderfully healing to the respiratory system. Mix a few drops of the essential oils or these herbs with one-quarter cup of **almond** or **apricot oil.** Massage this onto the chest, arms, and legs while taking a steambath. The steam will loosen up the lungs and open up the pores of the skin, allowing toxins to be released. Try to stay in the steam for 20 minutes, then cool off with a cold shower. This will close the pores and refresh the mind.

— **Exercise, but don't burn out before the "miracle" happens.** Nicotine affects the metabolism. As a matter of fact, smokers burn up to 10 percent more energy than do nonsmokers. For this reason, it's important to do something physical every day. Foot-pounding exercise at a gym isn't necessary. However, taking a walk, riding a bike, using the stairs instead of an elevator, going for a swim, or signing up for a modern dance or folk dance class will help push the metabolism up, exercise the lungs, and improve one's mental attitude. If a new nonsmoker has led a sedentary life for quite some time, it's very important to slowly begin an exercise regime and build up the intensity of physical activity over several months.

— **Make some environmental changes.** Pack up ashtrays for storage. New nonsmokers will also benefit from looking through photographs in photo albums or framed pictures in search of smoking pictures. While making an album of these photos of yourself smoking, you can affirm to yourself, "Yes, that was me, the old me. Although the cigarettes served me well, they're now hurting me. The new me deserves a smoke-free life." This affirmation should then be written on five sheets of paper. Put one on the bathroom mirror, another on the refrigerator, one near a favorite smoking area in the house, another on the dashboard of your car, and place the last one in a wallet or purse. Place the "smoking" photo album with the ashtrays for storage. Replace ashtrays with fresh flowers and green plants.

It's also extremely important to clean the stale cigarette smoke smell from drapes, clothes, and cars. One quick coat of paint will remove the smoke smell on walls. A light-scented **lemon** or **lavender herbal wash** can also be used on the walls, along with countertops, cupboards, and drawers. Ceilings are notorious collectors of smoke odor, along with fans and air filters. These need to be cleaned, painted, or replaced. Making homemade potpourri and placing dishes of this throughout the house, office, and so on, can add a great deal of serenity to the new smoke-free home.

— **When an individual decides to stop smoking, dreams about picking up the cigarette and deeply inhaling are very common.** Such dreams usually indicate the presence of stress in the waking world, and this tension must be addressed. Turning to your journal and asking the cigarettes seen in the dream, "Why are you here? What are you trying to protect me from? Why am I stressed?" can produce some very enlightening answers.

— **Spiritual considerations also need to be addressed.** Ask other nonsmokers for support. Connecting with others can promote spiritual healing. Telephoning one nonsmoker a day for the first month of abstinence can be useful in preventing a relapse. Visualizing a concept of God or a Higher Power, angels, guides, or the creative spiritual force within and asking for assistance in abstaining from smoking will provide relief to the new nonsmoker. If a craving to smoke hits an hour or two later, taking a moment to close the eyes and make the request for assistance again can prevent a backslide.

— **Develop activities that will help you release emotional stress.** Kickboxing, writing angry letters, hitting golf balls, weight lifting, shredding paper, pounding nails into a board, or screaming into a pillow are just a few of the methods the new nonsmoker can use to release anger. Yoga, meditation, prayer, a hot herbal bath, or deep-breathing exercises are activities that can reduce fear, panic, and anxiety. If necessary, join a support group for nonsmokers, or visit a therapist for several sessions to develop appropriate skills that will positively aid you in effectively processing anger and fear.

— **Alternative therapies have proven to be of great value for those who choose to "kick" the smoking habit.** In 1985, a control study investigating methods utilized to help people stop smoking was set up to compare the effectiveness of acupuncture therapy with nicotine gum. Interestingly, both were not only equally effective, but still continued to have an impact at one- and 13-month follow-ups. Acupuncture is based on traditional Chinese medicine, and it has a rich, long tradition. In China, acupuncture has been a primary mode of treatment for 5,000 years. Today, other methods beside needles are used to stimulate acupoints. Electro-acupuncture uses an extremely small electrical current to stimulate the acupoints, and this procedure is painless. For some individuals, hypnosis has proven to be useful. A good hypnotist can replace negative beliefs (the need for a cigarette) with positive beliefs (a smoke-free life, clean lungs, and elevated self-esteem) deep in the subconscious.

Nutritional and Herbal Support for New Nonsmokers

An important area of healing that many stop-smoking programs ignore is nutrition. Good nutrition plays a vital role in achieving a smoke-free lifestyle because what we eat can have a dramatic effect on the mind. The body is a very complex organism that is quite capable of healing itself, if we'll only listen to what it's saying. Unfortunately, most of us stopped listening a long time ago. Instead, we've tuned in to the advertising jingles of the fast-food market. By learning to reconnect with our bodies, we can begin to build a healthy, lifelong partnership with our physical self. As Moses Maimonides so wisely stated over 800 years ago, "The physician should not treat the ailment, but the patient who is suffering from it." We must change our attitudes with regard to how we're nourishing our bodies.

Aside from having a number of calming benefits, many herbs have nutritional properties. Herbal craft is a long and difficult study, but there are many remedies available to the layperson that are tried and true. If attention is not given to the physical state of the individual attempting to abstain from the powerful draw of nicotine, it will be difficult to make the psychological and lifestyle changes necessary for a complete healing. Both nutrition and herbology can greatly decrease the probability of relapse. With this in mind, it's time to begin investigating the nutritional needs of the individual who has stopped smoking cigarettes.

A large number of smokers fail to recognize that most cigarette-related illnesses are directly tied in to nutrition. The effects of smoking on nutrition are many, and it's important for the new nonsmoker to be aware of this fact. Smoking cigarettes suppresses the function of the immune system. A healthy immune system will readily go to battle against disease-causing microorganisms and then work double-time to assist the body in the healing process. The white blood cells are the key warriors within this system of complex interactions. These particular cells are the primary force that the body depends on when battling against disease in the body. If the immune system's army of white blood cells becomes diminished, the war against disease can quickly be lost.

Smoking destroys Vitamin C, and this particular nutrient is required "food," so to speak, for the white blood cells. If the white blood cells do not receive enough of this vitamin, the immune system is weakened. Once the immune system is weakened, the smoker is at risk for a host of illnesses.

Many smokers delude themselves into thinking that they're at less risk for illness if they smoke only low-tar or specially filtered cigarettes. Many cigarette manufacturers perpetuate this myth with glossy ad campaigns. From a nutritional point of view, these cigarettes are not any safer. Also, those individuals who puff away on cigars or pipes tend to believe they're better off than the average smoker. In actuality, one pipeful of tobacco is equal to two cigarettes, while a medium-sized cigar is as dangerous as three cigarettes. Even being around someone who smokes will deplete the nutritional state of the body. Basically, where there's smoke, there's illness. As a result, a good, solid, healthy diet with nutritional supplements is strongly suggested for the new nonsmoker.

Many individuals fear weight gain when they quit smoking. Some even decide to begin severely restricting their calories. From a health standpoint, this definitely isn't the time to start starving the body. Others may run to the physician in search of diet pills, shots, or a "new" fad diet to keep the pounds off. Such action can be just as dangerous as smoking. By utilizing the following nutritional guidelines, the new nonsmoker will begin reclaiming a healthy body. As Hippocrates said so brilliantly centuries ago, "A wise man should consider that health is the greatest of human blessings."

— **Follow the "Healthy Body, Well Mind" diet plan** found in the Appendix. This diet plan is very well rounded, highly nutritional, and satisfying to the taste buds. Now is not the time to try a fad diet of any kind. The body is trying to heal, and it can only do so with proper nutritional support.

— **If there is a need to lose weight, begin by cutting only 200 calories out of the diet.** Stick to this particular guideline for a year. The physical body has a locked-in "fat stuck point," and if the body is starved, it will believe it's in a famine. In an attempt to conserve energy, the metabolism of the body is lowered. Once dieting ends and the normal consumption of food begins, the weight will pile back on because the metabolism will stay at this low point. Also, it's important to remember that cigarette smoking causes calories to be burned. Once the smoker abstains from cigarettes, this, too, will cause the metabolism to automatically lower itself.

— Follow the **supplement suggestions** in Appendix II. Only increase the dosages of those vitamins discussed in the following guidelines. Take all other supplements as suggested.

— Increase the intake of **Vitamin C.** Vitamin C greatly enhances the immune system. Nutritionists suggest that initially, 10,000 mg of Vitamin C be taken daily to make up for the loss caused by years of cigarette smoking. Be sure this supplement is buffered and that it also contains bioflavonoids. Divide the above dose into three daily doses, and follow this regimen for one month. Then return to normal doses.

— Increase the intake of **natural beta-carotene** for one month. The body will take this nutrient and convert it into Vitamin A. Vitamin A is extremely necessary for the protection and repair of lung tissue. According to noted vitamin researcher Patricia Hausman, unlike Vitamin A supplements, natural beta-carotene does not have a toxicity level. Increasing dosages of natural beta-carotene to 50,000 IU daily will assist the lung tissue in healing.

(**Note:** If the new nonsmoker is diabetic, has hypothyroidism, or severe liver malfunctioning, an increase in natural beta-carotene may be necessary because these conditions impair the body's ability to convert this nutrient into Vitamin A. If unsure of the dosage, consult with a qualified holistic health-care provider.)

— Increase dosages of **Vitamin E** to 800 IU, and divide this into two doses. Be sure to take this vitamin with Vitamin C. Vitamin E is a powerful oxygen carrier, and it's needed for healing tissue and improving breathing. This vitamin is also a wonderful free-radical scavenger.

— Use **zinc lozenges.** Zinc is needed to repair lung tissue. Take one 15 mg lozenge five times a day, but do not exceed a total daily dose of 100 mg daily from all supplements.

— **Free amino acid complex** can be found at any health food store. This nutrient is also necessary for lung-tissue repair.

— **Calcium,** in combination with **magnesium,** has a wonderful calming effect on the nervous system. For the first several months of abstinence, calcium and magnesium dosages need to be increased. Take 2,000 mg of calcium and 1,000 mg of magnesium at bedtime. Aside from being necessary "bone food," this mineral combination acts as a nerve tonic, and it promotes a better night's sleep.

As mentioned earlier, herbal remedies can play a number of roles in healing the body and calming the mind. For the purposes of this chapter, herbs to increase the energy level, detoxify the body, increase the burning of body fat, calm the nerves, and soothe the respiratory function will be examined.

— **Energy level** can become a concern for the new nonsmoker, but have no fear, the world of herbs has several natural solutions. **Citrin** is a trademark name for an herbal remedy that can be used to burn fat. The herbal extract from the fruit of the *Garcinia cambogia* plant is believed not only to burn off body fat, but also to suppress the appetite. Unlike over-the-counter appetite suppressants or traditional medical diet pills, this particular remedy does not affect the nervous system, and it has no known side effects. Take as directed on the label.

— **Bladderwrack,** a flat, brownish-green seashore algae, appears to raise the metabolism, and research has shown that it's useful for reducing weight. This herb can be used in tea, as a tincture, or in capsule form.

(**Note:** Do note take this herb if pregnant or breast-feeding. If suffering from a thyroid condition, take only under the advice of a professional.)

— Many smokers suffer from "smoker's cough." The hairy herb **mullein** can take care of this problem. Not only is this funny-looking plant a wonderful remedy for coughs, but at one time, Roman women used to make a blonde hair wash with it. Steeped as a tea, this herb is noted for its value as a cough medicine.

(**Note:** Remember to strain the tea to keep the small hairs of this plant from irritating the throat.)

Also, a decoction of **slippery elm** and **wild cherry bark** (made by boiling the dried ingredients in a minimal amount of water) will soothe the throat and silence a hacking cough.

— The herb **fenugreek** has a lot to offer the new nonsmoker. Aside from its history of usage as a breast-enlargement treatment for women in harems in North Africa and the Middle East, this herb is recommended as a remedy by herbalists for reducing excessive bronchial mucus. Another herb to consider for the bronchial area is **horsetail.** Although this herb was at one time tied to the tails of livestock to ward off insects, today it's known for its anti-inflammatory properties and its ability to reduce dry coughing. Both of these herbs can be used in an infusion.

(**Note:** Do not use fenugreek if pregnant, and do not use horsetail for more than six weeks. Do not confuse horsetail with the toxic marsh horsetail plant.)

— The **garlic bulb** has a rich folklore tradition. In times past, not only was this particular smelly herb carried by new brides to bring them love and luck in their new marriage, but it was placed under children's pillows to protect them from the evils of the night. Taken regularly in capsule form, garlic can aid in detoxing the body, lowering blood pressure and cholesterol levels, thinning the blood, reducing bronchial mucus, and fighting infection. A great deal of research has been done on this herb, and the results have been overwhelmingly positive. When the smoker puts down the cigarette, initially the nerves will seem frayed. As the repressed emotions of anger and fear come screaming to the surface, the new nonsmoker initially will wonder if giving up the smokes was such a good idea. Once again, the knowledge of the well-trained herbalist can come to the rescue. The sweet-smelling herb **lemon balm** has long been used to chase away melancholy and lift the spirits. This herb can reduce panic attacks; and relieve mild depression, irritability, nervousness, and heart palpitations. The herb with the palm-shaped leaves and pink flowers traditionally considered as a heart remedy is known as **motherwort**. This pretty herb acts as a gentle sedative, and it promotes relaxation without drowsiness. (**Note:** Do not use this herb if pregnant or during heavy menstrual bleeding.)

The yellow-flowered herb **damiana** used by Mexican women as a sexual aphrodisiac is also useful for mild depression and anxiety. For mild depression, take any of the above herbal remedies in a tincture form.

— The Native American herb **lobelia** or "puke weed" (this herb is also used to induce vomiting), has pale blue flowers that were once thought to ward off ghosts. Aside from tormenting the spirit world, this particular herb has been used as a substitute for tobacco. Lobelia is chemically similar to nicotine. If the smoker chooses to use this herb, it's important that he or she do so under the guidance of a qualified herbalist.

By implementing the above psychology, lifestyle, and nutritional/herbal changes, the new nonsmoker will begin to reap the rewards of a smoke-free life.

Shelly looked closely at her friends and smiled. "You two look great."

With this, Elizabeth replied, "And I feel great. Putting the cigarettes down was a challenge, but I like the way I feel and look. Did you know that cigarette smoke ages the skin prematurely? That did it for me. I'm much too vain to allow a little stick of tobacco to wreck my skin."

Joyce took a sip of her iced green tea. Then she said, "When I quit smoking, all of this rage suddenly appeared from out of the blue. At first I thought I was losing my mind."

Shelly grabbed a piece of garlic bread from the basket and replied, "Really? You experienced rage? What on earth did you do about it?"

With a wicked smile, Joyce proudly announced, "I finally put it where it belonged. I used my newfound rage to put closure on my relationship with my ex-husband. Every time this emotion overwhelmed me, I visualized him and said all of the things I was never able to say before. Then I put it in a letter and mailed it. And I feel great."

Elizabeth leaned over, embraced Joyce, and with joy, replied, "Geez, girl. It's about time. Now maybe you can move on with your life!"

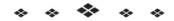

Chapter thirteen

ADDICTIVE BEHAVIOR: HIDING FROM LIFE WITH ALCOHOL AND DRUGS

D r. Levy looked at his watch. Time was slipping away. He had spent the morning at home on the phone talking with a patient, a recovering alcoholic who had called with a question about "drunk dreams." Dr. Levy assured the frantic voice on the other end of the line that dreams about drinking were very normal in early sobriety.

As Dr. Levy loaded up his car with house paint, he thought to himself, *Where is the painter?* Dr. Levy's office was housed in a 100-year-old historical property, and it was in need of a new paint job. The Cinderella-looking house was nestled between two large magnolia trees, and nobody would have ever suspected that it served as a mental health facility for recovering alcoholics and drug addicts.

As he rummaged through his briefcase, Dr. Levy asked his wife, "Where the heck is he? If I don't get going, I'm going to miss my first appointment." His wife gave him a gentle pat on the back and replied, "Well, I guess this is my fault. I was told that this painter is great—when he shows up for work. From what I hear, he hardly ever makes it to a job on Monday mornings. You and I both know what that means."

Dr. Levy knew exactly what that meant. For a number of years, he, too, had a hard time getting to the office after a weekend of beer, wine coolers, and tranquilizers. His head always felt four times its size. Looking at his wife, he asked, "Do you think that the painter might have a problem with alcohol or drugs?" With this, she laughed out loud and then said, "Duh."

For years I, too, thought I was just weak and lacking in willpower. During my decade of serious drinking, I switched from hard liquor to beer and then wine, but my hangovers didn't improve. Because I only took what the doctor gave me, I also never believed I was a drug addict. Years later, I had to admit that I wasn't very truthful with my doctor about the number of other pills I was taking. The combination of tranquilizers and alcohol almost killed me, but in spite of this, I continued to drink. For some time, I suffered from a very deadly disease and didn't even know it.

Out of 38 active chemically dependent persons—those addicted to alcohol, drugs, or both—only one will achieve a sober lifestyle. One out of every three families in this country is directly affected by alcohol and drug addiction. Currently, it's estimated that these addictions affect at least ten million people in the United States and are responsible for 200,000 deaths each year. Alcoholism, and addiction to illegal or prescription drugs, is a genetic condition that crosses all cultural and economic barriers. Several years ago, the gene for alcoholism was isolated. If one has inherited this particular gene from a parent, grandparent, uncle, aunt, or cousin, this person, too, is at risk for developing the disease of chemical dependence.

Just what does a chemically dependent person look like? When most of us picture an alcoholic or addict, we usually think of a street bum, living on a corner or under a bridge. Although such individuals may be chemically dependent, most afflicted with this disease look just like you and me. They have intact families, jobs, a car, a home, and even a responsible position within society. They are male, female, young, old, white, brown, black, and yellow. Some of them are daily users of drugs and alcohol, while others use these chemicals only on weekends. With all of these differences, how are these people alike?

First of all, there are always consequences to their use of drugs or alcohol, and these consequences can impact every area of life. In spite of lost jobs, destroyed marriages, drunk-driving charges, health difficulties, lost dreams and goals, disconnected spiritual lives, financial issues, and difficult relations with children and other family members, a person plagued with chemical dependence will not put down the drink, joint, pill, line, or needle. Such individuals have great difficulty seeing that the negative consequences of their life are directly tied to the use of drugs and alcohol. Second, family members, friends, or acquaintances on the job usually have a concern about an alcoholic or addict's chemical use, but they rarely connect this to physical, emotional, social, legal, or spiritual difficulties.

Yes, this is a frightening illness. In my years of experience, I've found that long-term recovery from chemical dependence is only possible when a holistic approach is applied. For healing to take hold, all aspects of the person must be addressed. Before the psychology behind this condition can be contemplated, certain lifestyle changes must be made.

Essential Lifestyle Changes for the Chemically Dependent Person

For the chemically dependent person, the first drink swallowed or drug ingested will set off the compulsion to continue to consume alcohol or use mood-altering substances. Once this compulsion is in play, it's difficult to determine:

- how much of the mood altering chemical will be consumed in one sitting, and
- the consequences of the ingestion of the chemical.

Although many chemically dependent persons suffer regularly from their use of alcohol or drugs, most can go for months without experiencing consequences. Eventually, control is lost and consequences are suffered. In either case, the outcome can be devastating.

The lifestyle behind this disease is often ignored by traditional mental-health caregivers. Instead, such professionals tend to look at personal problems as the instigators of excessive alcohol or drug use. Little do they understand that many of the current difficulties with relationships, self-esteem, depression, and more are a direct result of alcohol and drug-using behavior. Before emotional, physical, or spiritual healing can begin, the drinking of alcohol or use of drugs must be addressed.

— **"The first drink or drug will get you in trouble"** is a phrase often repeated by many recovering alcoholics and addicts. A non-addicted person is able to periodically have one or two drinks or even "tie one on," without suffering major consequences, but a problem drinker is not so lucky. The same is true for drug use. For the chemically dependent person, the first drink or hit sets off a physical desire for more of the chemical. I believe that chemical dependence is similar to a food allergy. A person who's addicted to a particular substance, in this case drugs or alcohol, craves more of that substance even though it isn't healthy for them.

How do you determine whether you have a problem with mood-altering substances? Give yourself permission to have one drink, joint, pill, or whatever your substance of choice is, every day for six months. See what happens. Do you crave more? Drink or use more? Black out?

(**Note:** One who experiences a blackout or loss of memory after ingesting mood-altering chemicals can look very normal to those around them. If you've had a blackout, you might have an addiction to contend with.)

— **Support.** Once it's determined that ingesting chemicals is a problem, abstinence can feel impossible. Support groups such as Alcoholics Anonymous, Cocaine Anonymous, Pills Anonymous, or Narcotics Anonymous can be of great aid. These meetings are free of charge and have helped millions of people around the world. To find a meeting in your area, call the main office for Alcoholics Anonymous in New York at (212) 870-3400, or look in the yellow pages of your telephone directory. When you go to your first meeting, they will ask if there's anyone attending the meeting for the first time. If you feel uncomfortable responding, remain silent but continue to attend five more times. Listen to what is being said. Don't compare your drug or alcohol history with those speaking at the meeting. Instead, focus in on the feelings that are being expressed. Listen to how the members of the group have resolved some of their life difficulties. After six visits, if you feel you don't fit in with this group, find another meeting and attend it six times. Meeting with others who have had difficulty abstaining from the first drink or drug can assist you in achieving sobriety. If these particular groups don't work for you, call the alcohol and drug helpline at 1-800-ALCOHOL for information on other groups.

— **If you want to quit using drugs and alcohol, give yourself a break.** During the early days of sobriety, avoiding places where alcohol is readily available is essential. Why make yourself miserable by putting yourself in situations where alcohol will be right there, in your face. Does this mean that you need to become a hermit who isolates yourself from the joy of living? Heavens, no! You can have gatherings at your home. Instead of liquor, serve an assortment of flavored coffees, teas, or even milkshakes. Create new traditions for yourself. Invite friends over to play games, cook a feast, or view movies. You *can* continue to have fun in life. Just make sure you're sober when you do so.

I have been sober, off prescription drugs and alcohol, for many years. Today, I can be around alcohol without feeling compelled to pick up a drink. If there's a lot of drinking going on, I quickly become bored. With sobriety, I've learned to appreciate clear-headed conversations. Trying to talk to someone who's intoxicated is no fun at all. The ability to enjoy life without alcohol came with time, so for the first few days, weeks, months, and even years of sobriety, give yourself a break. Stay away from places where alcohol and drugs rule the party.

— **Exercise.** Addiction to drugs and alcohol can leave us out of touch with the physical body. For several years, I spent time working with chemically dependent young teens. One of these young people desperately wanted to learn how to surf. Unfortunately, his obsession with alcohol kept him from achieving this goal. After a few weeks of abstinence, he decided to take his board out to the ocean and give it a try. Today, when I travel up and down the oceanfront near my home, I often see him riding the waves. As he said to me several years later, "Surfing gives me a high I never knew I could achieve naturally."

Make a list of all of the physical activities you'd like to try. Pick an activity, but don't push yourself or your body. Excessive alcohol and drug use puts tremendous stress on the body. Build up your strength slowly.

— **Education will make you feel sane.** When I decided to begin a sober life, I took a class on how addiction had not only affected me, but also those I loved. The class served several purposes. First, chatting with other people suffering from addictions helped me understand my disease. Seeing men and women from all walks of life grappling with this illness helped me realize that I was not in this battle all by myself.

Second, understanding the physiology of my compulsion to use mood-altering chemicals proved to me that I really was dealing with a true biological illness. Third, numerous family members of chemically dependent people were in attendance at this class. I learned that addiction impacts every member of a family for several generations. This information gave me a better perspective on my own alcoholic parents. As I listened to the lectures on chemical dependence and the family, it became clear that I had been destined to become drug and alcohol addicted. Learning this particular fact increased my desire to break the cycle. Finally, knowing that my disease had hurt my family was extremely painful, but it helped me become even more committed to my own healing process. Since taking this class, I've been with groups of chemically dependent people who are also astronauts, athletes, movie stars, rock stars, housewives, lawyers, college students, doctors, bankers, military personnel, and even young children.

The Psychology of Chemical Dependency

— **Before anything, one month of sobriety first.** It's impossible to resolve psychological issues if alcohol or drugs continues to be ingested by a chemically dependent person. In my private practice, I will see such a person for only five sessions. During this time, I provide them with resources and support for getting sober. After five sessions, if an attempt at sobriety has not been made, I will say, "This is a waste of your money and my time. As long as you retreat to alcohol or drugs, we will never be able to work through the emotions you carry regarding current and past difficulties. Blunting your emotions with mood-altering chemicals distances you from the feelings you need to be processing to heal." (This is why I placed the lifestyle section of this book ahead of the psychology section.)

After abstinence has been achieved and sobriety has been maintained for a month, it's possible to begin examining a few of the psychological issues perpetuating the alcoholism or drug addiction.

— **Unresolved grief issues.** Unresolved grief issues usually facilitate alcoholic drinking or drug use in those individuals who carry the gene for this disease. You might be asking yourself, "Why is this?" The reason is that grief issues are not totally embraced by the American culture. As a result, mental health is often determined by how quickly one rebounds from trauma or loss. There are other cultures that encourage the expression of strong emotions, but sadly, ours is not on this list. This cultural fact can actually perpetuate chemical dependence, especially in those who carry the gene for this illness.

For the chemically dependent individual, avoiding the pain of a loved one's death; or dealing with lost relationships, financial disappointments, a traumatic childhood, unfulfilled dreams, a job change, divorce, a severe illness, and a host of other life disappointments can facilitate drinking or drugging. The day my mother died, I picked up my first drink. I was only 16 years old and desperately wanted the pain to go away. For several years, alcohol numbed the anguish I carried with respect to a number of losses. At the age of 27, I quit drinking and had to honestly face these losses, one at a time, over a period of years.

So, make a list of all of your life disappointments. Include everything, even if you believe that something no longer affects you. Acknowledging these losses is the first step of the psychological healing process.

— **Learning how to feel.** Learning how to fully feel these losses is the second step in healing emotionally from chemical dependence. Most chemically dependent individuals are frightened of their emotions, especially intense feelings of rage, terror, and grief. Feeling comfortable with these emotions does take time, so it's important for you to be gentle with yourself.

The following exercise can be done slowly, over a period of months: Discuss each of your losses with a therapist or spiritual advisor, or write a letter of sadness about this to your higher self, your guardian angel, or your concept of God or a Higher Power. Remember, requesting help is not a sign of weakness; it's a show of strength.

As mentioned earlier, excessive drug and alcohol use affects the body, mind, and soul. We've examined what it is we must do to heal the mind. Now let's take a look at what the body needs.

Nutritional and Herbal Support for "New Sobriety"

Because alcoholic beverages tend to be high in sugar, the nutritional state of a newly sober person can be frightening. When involved in the disease of chemical dependence, a healthy diet is not a top priority. Since alcohol raises blood-sugar levels, when a chemically dependent person decides to sober up, this can throw the body's blood-sugar balance into chaos. Also, the physical body has been starved of nutrients—in some cases, for many, many years. Depending on the severity of the addiction and the number of years involved in the disease, physical consequences to alcohol or drug use can include liver and heart damage; possible high blood pressure; and a higher risk for breast cancer, stroke, stomach problems, mouth cancer, ulcers, kidney difficulties, impotence, pancreatitis, premature aging, and esophagus cancer. The central nervous system can also be dramatically affected by excessive drug or alcohol use. Leg cramps, along with numbness in the extremities, is not uncommon.

It's always interesting to see how intertwined the body and mind are. With chemical dependence, this connection is very apparent. As we are learning, any nutrient deficiency can dramatically impact mental functioning. Getting the physical body "up to snuff" will dramatically improve the mood of the newly sober person.

— **Start out simply.** For at least a month, the mind will be foggy. As a result, it's important to keep nutritional supplementation simple. Begin by taking a trip to a reputable health food store. Ask for an organically based, high-potency multivitamin. Make sure your supplement is one that is easily absorbed by the system. Use Appendix II as your guideline. The key terms here are *high-potency* and *easily absorbed.*

— **Look out for hypoglycemia.** This is a blood-sugar condition. As mentioned earlier, excessive alcohol use can leave blood-sugar levels out of balance. Hypoglycemia is common in newly sober people. It also contributes to a poor mental state and increased withdrawal symptoms, leaving one feeling depressed, shaky, dizzy, anxious, confused, and overwhelmed. **Spirulina,** a "green food," is full of nutrients necessary for a balanced blood-sugar level. Personally, I think the stuff tastes just awful, so I recommend using this food supplement in tablet form. At the health food store, you'll find various brands of spirulina. Choose one that is not only organic and pure, but pesticide free. Take as directed on the label. The mineral **chromium** can assist in leveling out "haywire" blood-sugar levels. This nutrient is also believed to reduce the sugar cravings that often accompany the detoxification process in newly sober people. The suggested dose for alcohol or drug withdrawal is 200 micrograms of chromium once or twice a day.

— **Nutritional rescue for cell damage.** Addiction leads to damaged cells, and damaged cells mean poor health. Vitamins with antioxidant properties can repair the havoc that alcohol and drugs create on the structure of the cells. Begin by increasing Vitamin C levels. Your total intake of **Vitamin C** per day should be 3,000 mg. Divide this into three separate doses. For those in early sobriety, it's suggested that 400 IU of **Vitamin E** be taken twice a day. Vitamin E will protect blood cells and assist in increasing endurance by supplying more oxygen to the body.

(**Note:** Do not take Vitamin E if you're on blood-thinning anticoagulant medication.)

— **Don't forget the Bs.** Vitamin B deficiency is extremely common with chemical dependence. This deficiency often accounts for the tremors and shakes that newly sober men and women experience during chemical withdrawal. Take an organically based **Vitamin B complex** tablet every day.

— **Help for the liver.** The liver is responsible for metabolizing toxins. When the liver is overworked, it begins to suffer damage in the form of hepatitis, cirrhosis, fatty degeneration, and cancer. Taking 250 to 500 mg of the amino acid **L-carnitine** with breakfast will begin to repair any liver damage. After taking this dose for a week, add a second daily dose at lunchtime. In the third week, begin taking an added dose of L-carnitine at dinnertime. It's suggested that this regimen continue for three to four months. Give the liver another boost with 500 mg of the mineral **choline,** and 500 mg of the amino acid **gluthione** twice a day. Your liver will thank you. Be sure to check dosages in your multivitamin before supplementing with choline, gluthione, or L-carnitine.

— **Sleep tight.** Taking 300 mg of **magnesium** and 1,500 mg of **calcium** just before bed will ensure a restful sleep.

A balanced diet rich in fruits, vegetables, lean meats, fish, low-fat dairy products, and whole grains—while low in white refined sugar and saturated fats—is also necessary for nutritional health. Fresh vegetable juices such as carrot are not only nutritious, but also full of Vitamin A, which is essential for healthy liver function. Along with carrots, throw a handful of parsley into your juicer. Parsley is a great blood purifier. Once nutritional deficiencies are rectified, the state of the body will improve. How often I've heard, "I never knew I could feel this great!" from sober individuals who have taken the time to repair their nutritional state. Let's see what we can gather for healing, herb-wise. Once again, we return to the liver.

— **Milk thistle** is a very pretty plant. When the flower is in bloom, it's bright pink. This particular herb has been used for centuries by Europeans. Milk thistle has the ability to metabolize the fat that tends to accumulates in the liver of chemically dependent people. This herb can be used in tea or capsule form. Use as directed.

— **Red clover** makes a nice tea, but when combined with **burdock root, dandelion root,** and **yellow dock,** it becomes part of a powerful herbal remedy. All of the above herbs have a purifying effect on the body and are useful during detoxification from drugs or alcohol. Take one teaspoon of burdock root and dandelion root, and place in a stainless steel pan. Pour two cups of water over this mixture. Bring to a boil, and then simmer until half of the liquid has evaporated. Take the mixture off of the stove and add one tea bag of yellow dock, red clover, and peppermint (for flavor), and then cover. Steep for 20 minutes. Strain the liquid from the herbs, and add four cups of water. Sweeten with honey, refrigerate, and drink two ounces, three times a day.

— **Let's talk about stress.** New sobriety can be very stressful. Viewing the world from a newly sober perspective can rattle the mind and the body. According to Greek myth, the nymph Philya was turned into a **linden** tree. The poor girl had been raped by the god Saturn, who at the time was disguised as a horse. She later gave birth to a famous centaur, but the experience was so traumatic that she begged the gods not to ever leave her with mortals. As a linden tree, she was well disguised.

In early sobriety, I suffered from anxiety and nervous heart palpitations. Linden is a wonderful herb for these conditions. In addition, linden will calm the mind and assist us in slipping into a restful sleep at night. Check your local health food store for linden flower tops in tea form or capsules. Use as directed.

When one decides to take a sober path, the challenges on the road are great, but the rewards can be enormous. If you have a problem with drugs or alcohol, know that you're not alone. You deserve all of the joy that sobriety has to offer.

Dr. Levy had just finished with his last patient for the day. As he escorted her out the door, he noticed that the painter was washing out his brushes. Waving good-bye to his patient, he turned to the painter and asked, "Are you ready to go?"

"Yep," the blond-haired man replied.

Once in the car, the painter turned to Dr. Levy and asked, "Do you think I might have a problem with alcohol?"

With this, Dr. Levy responded, "I can't tell you whether or not you're an alcoholic. That's something you will have to figure out for yourself. If you're concerned about your drinking, you might want to educate yourself on the disease of chemical dependence. Hey, I was planning on going to an AA meeting after I dropped you off. Why don't you join me?"

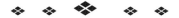

PART VI

Loving—and Leaving—Food

❧ ❧ ❧ ❧

Chapter fourteen

OBSESSIVE-COMPULSIVE EATING

Sherry was so excited. It was her first Caribbean cruise. As she walked the halls of the ship, she wondered where her husband, Gary, had gone. Stepping out onto the pool deck, she saw a pretty woman coming through the door. *Gee, look at her!* Sherry sighed. The attractive middle-aged woman was wearing a brightly colored bathing suit. Sherry's eyes followed her as she made her way to stairs, leading to a lower deck. *Now why can't I look like that?!* she thought angrily.

After searching the pool deck for Gary, Sherry decided to check the lunchroom. Wearing the loudest Hawaiian shirt in the room, her husband wasn't hard to spot. The bright colors ran together and clashed terribly with his checked shorts. A shock of red hair was escaping a Boston Red Sox baseball cap. *He looks like a true tourist. All he needs is a camera hanging around his neck, and the picture would be complete,* thought Sherry.

Gary had found a table and was already enjoying a forkful of cheesy potatoes. Every food item that he had taken from the buffet was either full of fat or had been fried. After the potatoes, he went for a bit of macaroni salad. Sherry sat down, picked up a spoon, and also dug into the mayonnaise-soaked macaroni. "Oh, that's divine! Hey, is that fried chicken on your platter?

Yummy. Let me have a piece," she demanded.

Gary grabbed his plate away from her, smiled, and said, "I thought we were going to watch what we eat on this trip."

As she made another attempt to grab his chicken, Sherry replied, "Very funny."

One third of the adult American population is seriously overweight. Excessive weight gain increases the risk of coronary artery disease, diabetes, gall bladder disease; high blood pressure, kidney disease and stroke; stress on the legs, back, and internal organs; susceptibility to infection; and a host of other illnesses. Sadly, the overweight person can't hide the extra pounds he or she carries. This, in turn, compounds already existing psychological pain for the overweight individual.

The Psychology of Obsessive-Compulsive Eating

Although many "quick weight-loss" programs contend that excessive body weight has more to do with physical factors than emotional issues, the psychology behind compulsive eating can't be ignored. Compulsive eating is a mood-altering behavior, and some foods can actually change the body chemistry. Children often learn at an early age that certain foods will medicate strong emotions. As an eight-year-old told me, "Sugar makes me feel better." During moments of stress, kids will continue to reach for those particular foods.

This behavior can carry over into adult life. When this happens, compulsive eating becomes a survival skill. On a short-term basis, this behavior is most effective in blocking strong emotions. Sadly, the long-term consequences eventually serve as a distraction from major life issues. Feeling obsessed and depressed about how one looks in the mirror provides a great diversion from much of the emotional pain, loss, disappointment, or trauma that life often offers up. Along with yo-yo dieting, obsessing on food or diets is an extremely effective distancing mechanism. Yes, obsessive-compulsive eating does serve a psychological purpose and, no, diets do not cure the obsession. Excessive consumption of the wrong types of food is just one piece of a much larger puzzle. There are many other segments to this condition that must be addressed. The whole person must be treated to ensure complete, lifelong healing.

— **Fat is not the enemy.** For most compulsive eaters, fat has been seen as the enemy. "When I lose this weight, my life will finally turn around," is what I have heard over and over again from compulsive eaters. Recognizing that compulsive eating has a purpose is essential. Emotional medication with food keeps anger, depression, fear, and other more destructive behaviors at a distance. As long as I'm focused on my weight and am berating myself for being too heavy, I don't have to confront any of the hurts of my present or past.

For those of us who haven't developed healthy tools for living, compulsive eating serves as a survival skill. If someone harms me emotionally or physically and I don't know how to confront this issue, I can fall back on what has worked in the past. That just might be a bag of chocolate chip cookies, a handful of greasy chips, or too much food at dinnertime. By numbing our feelings with food, the experience of being hurt is temporarily repressed. It's important to understand that this survival skill is not the enemy. It originated for a reason. Here is a visualization that will help clarify this concept:

Visualize your excessive weight. Maybe this image will be an ice cream cone or a wall of fat. Next, imagine yourself apologizing to this image. That's right. This survival skill has been protecting you. Thank this survival skill for being there for you during times of stress. Understand that without this survival skill, you may have self-destructed with even more damaging behaviors. Write about your experience with this visualization on a separate piece of paper.

— **Trigger feelings.** As mentioned earlier, food medicates the emotions. White sugar, overprocessed foods, and greasy meals can be especially mood-altering. When I was a child, my grandmother comforted me with a number of homemade luscious, rich, fatty, baked foods. In adulthood, these nurturing treats became my trigger foods. If stressed, angry, or sad, I would unconsciously run to my comfort foods. Every one of us has certain trigger foods. For some, it's chocolate, while for others, it's onion dip and potato chips.

It's important to recognize how our current comfort foods may be directly tied into many of the foods we loved as children. Most of us don't eat just one chip—we eat the whole bag. A small slice of cake or lasagna is never satisfying. Yes, we will eat until we feel nurtured.

On a separate sheet of paper, list your favorite foods. Put a red star next to those foods you compulsively eat or binge on. Next, place a green star by the foods you enjoyed as a child. Now circle all of the foods on your list that have a green and red star next to them. These are your trigger foods.

In the future, when we find ourselves compulsively eating these foods, we can ask, "Why am I so in need of nurturing? Am I sad, depressed, or feeling alone? Has someone recently hurt my feelings? Am I angry about something?" Looking at compulsive eating in this light clearly shows how food has served us as a protective mechanism.

— **Take care of the emotions, and process them out.** Life is full of bumps, bangs, and temporary bruises. The hard times will always come again, but must we continue to medicate with food to survive? Learning how to express grief, intense rage, the pain of shame, or the overwhelming sensation of terror can be life-saving. A therapist who uses experiential therapeutic techniques can teach you how to dump intense emotions. Also, involvement in support groups, spiritual guidance, or other self-help activities can assist you in learning how to manage your feelings. If you don't learn how to move through your emotions, you'll end up stuffing them with food. And stuffing your emotions with food will pile on the pounds.

Psychological difficulties cannot be totally resolved if lifestyle issues are ignored. For those who suffer from compulsive eating, loneliness can be prevalent. This is especially true if food has become a reward, punishment, lover, companion, and friend. Once it's realized that food can no longer play such a powerful role in your life, this must be filled with live, loving companions. In order to achieve this goal, lifestyle issues need to be examined.

Lifestyle Remedies for Healing Obsessive-Compulsive Eating

— Break out of *isolation*. Isolation emotionally starves a lonely soul, and this, in turn, can widen the waistline. Learning how to engage in "small talk" may initially sound like a total waste of time, but it isn't. Before we can have healthy intimacy with others, we have to develop friendships. In order to have friends, it's helpful to first have acquaintances. If we want to have acquaintances, it's important to learn how to talk to people. Recovery programs such as Overeaters Anonymous, Adult Children of Alcoholics Anonymous, or Co-dependents Anonymous can provide safe environments to begin learning how to do so. Church groups, spiritual study groups, meditation groups, art organizations, music companies, pet clubs, neighborhood associations, historical foundations, and garden clubs are also helpful.

— **Exercise.** Most compulsive eaters have led a sedentary lifestyle for some time. If your health-care provider has given you the "thumbs up" to begin exercising, it's time to dig out those sweat pants. Physical activity will begin to improve low metabolism, a common by-product of excessive weight. Do not jump into a rigorous high-impact exercise program. Instead, start slowly. Begin with a few simple changes in everyday living. Before going to work, during lunch or after dinner, take a short walk around the block. Use the stairs instead of the elevator. Whenever it's necessary to pick up a few groceries at the store, ride a bicycle. In order for exercise to be effective, it should be enjoyable. If it feels too "punishing," the desire to stick with it will quickly evaporate. Explore a variety of lively activities such as dance, swimming, rowing, weight lifting, hiking, gardening, or any other activity requiring physical effort. Daily exercise will burn up calories, increase your metabolic rate, and calm your mind.

— **Remove the whole idea of dieting from your consciousness.** As I said earlier, diets do not work. They are a total waste of time, money, and emotional energy. Once you stop following a particular fad diet, the weight will return. Most compulsive eaters have been on a variety of diets. Weight is lost and then the metabolism drops. The metabolism drops because there's less energy (food) to burn. The body learns to function on less energy. Once the diet ends and normal eating is resumed, the metabolism doesn't immediately return to a higher level. As a result, weight is then gained. Avoid fad diets, even those endorsed by celebrities. It's essential to understand that good nutrition doesn't mean dieting.

Nutrition and Herbs for Recovery from Obsessive-Compulsive Eating

In working with compulsive eaters, I have found that many sufferers are in a deplorable nutritional state. Most compulsive eaters need a great deal of education about healthy eating. After having survived on a diet of nutritionally void foods, this is extremely important. Without addressing the nutritional issues associated with this condition, doing work in the area of psychology and lifestyle is pointless.

— **A food journal** is essential. Let's honestly take a look at what is going into the body. Chances are it's a lot of nutritionally empty food. If you're vitamin deficient, how can you possibly be in a healthy mental place to process out psychological traumas and make major lifestyle changes? It just won't happen. This is why a food journal is so necessary, especially in the early phases of the healing process. A food journal provides two important pieces of information.

First of all, by documenting all that is eaten every day for two weeks, several things will be discovered:

- The makeup of the diet
- Meals skipped (breakfast jump starts the metabolism and is often skipped by compulsive eaters)
- Addictive foods (such as sugar, dairy products, wheat-baked foods, etc.)
- Trigger foods (which set off bingeing patterns)
- Mood-altering foods (excessive sugar, food additives, white flour, salts)

The journal will also reveal *high-risk* times of the day, those periods when compulsive eating is most likely to occur.

In addition, the food journal will begin to identify what type of life stresses facilitate binge behavior or compulsive eating. For example, Lisa maintains a very healthy food plan until it's time for her to go home to her husband, Bob. Once home, Lisa knows that Bob will begin to drink his six-pack of beer. Lisa doesn't know how to process her anger, hurt, and fear about Bob's drinking. As a result, Lisa finds that the more Bob drinks, the more she binges on trigger foods.

Identifying binge periods or times during the day when unhealthy food is consumed is another by-product of the food journal. The food journal can provide a wealth of information if food intake is honestly listed. Without truthfulness, the food journal will prove to be useless.

— **Education.** What does an excessive amount of white sugar do to the body? Sugar in any form will trigger the release of insulin. Insulin will then activate those enzymes that increase the movement of fat from the bloodstream into the fat cells. Yikes! Sugar helps build up fat cells.

And what about those diet sodas? Here is another source of empty calories that will create havoc in the body. Caffeine stimulates the appetite. Caffeinated diet sodas can make one hungry. Also, if the diet consists of too many nutritionally deficient foods, the body will continue to feel hungry because it craves nutrition. How about "light" beer and other alcoholic drinks? Exchanging the healthy calories in nutritional food for the empty calories in alcohol slows down the body's ability to burn off fat. Yes, nutritional education makes it difficult to munch down on unhealthy foods without thinking twice about the consequences. Ignorance is no longer bliss.

— **Baby steps.** Give each of the following steps a month to settle into your lifestyle and then move on to the next:

- Start by consuming **six to eight cups of liquid** (not sodas, but herbal teas, water, or vegetable juices) per day.

- Next, replace fatty foods with **complex carbohydrates.** Calories from fatty foods are easily converted into body fat. Only 3 percent of the fat calories ingested from such foods are burned by the digestive process. Instead of fried chicken or fried fish, try eating more pastas, lean meats, fish, potatoes, rice, and whole grains. Experiment with fruit salads, vegetables, and low-fat dairy products. During the digestive process, 25 percent of the calories from complex carbohydrates are burned.

- Loving yourself includes taking the time to **prepare nutritious, health-conscious meals.** Take a cooking class or experiment with low-fat cookbooks. A healthy diet doesn't need to be bland and boring. Learn how to cook, and then take the time to do so.

- **S-L-O-W-L-Y eliminate trigger foods** from your diet. Because this is such a major change, don't eliminate all trigger foods at once. Do this slowly. If Mom's coconut cream pie is the one food that really gets the binge ball rolling, you'll need to eliminate it from your diet. After a month or two, take a look at your second most powerful trigger food and decide when you'll begin abstaining from it.

(**Note:** This is a grief issue. Saying good-bye to foods that have helped you through stressful times can bring up many strong feelings. Don't ignore or stuff your sadness.)

— It's *extremely important* for you to respect your body's **fat set point.** The fat set point is a particular body weight. Your body has a comfortable fat set point, and your metabolism is adjusted to this. If you reduce your intake of calories too quickly, your body will think it's in a famine, and your metabolism will drop. You don't want this to happen. This is why diets never work. It's important not to reduce your caloric intake by more than 200 calories at a time. After creating your food journal, try to *honestly* calculate how many calories you're consuming on a weekly basis.

Once you've calculated this total, divide it by seven. You'll now have an approximation of your caloric intake for the day. Subtract 200 calories from this number. You will now have the approximate number of calories you need to ingest each day to maintain your body's fat set point. Stick to this calorie count for the next month. The following month, you may drop 200 more calories from your diet. Remember, balancing the body is the goal of a good nutritional program, not rapid weight loss. Slowly, over time, movement can be made toward removing more excess pounds.

— **Supplements.** The nutritionally starved body of the obsessive-compulsive eater can always benefit from vitamins and minerals in the form of supplements. By supplementing a slow-changing diet (moving from unhealthy, nutritionally bankrupt foods to a more complete nutritional program) with the vitamins and minerals necessary for health, success can be just around the corner. Follow the **Supplement for Health Program** found in Appendix II. Below is a list of additional nutrient supplements that should be considered:

- **Chromium picolinate**—400 mcg per day. This will reduce cravings for sugar.
- **Kelp**—Take as directed. This aids in weight loss.
- **Lecithin**—1,200 mg three times per day. This nutrient

will help break down fat so that it can be removed from the body.

- **Vitamin C**—3,000–6,000 mg divided into three doses per day. This wonderful vitamin will help speed up metabolism so it can burn up more calories.

- **Spirulina tablets**—Take between meals as directed. This will stabilize the blood sugar, and it contains a great deal of nutrients.

Before we leave this section, we need to talk about herbs. Instead of soda pop, brew up some raspberry, mandarin orange, peppermint, apple, cinnamon, lemon, or apricot tea, and put it on ice. When the desire to compulsively eat hits, pour yourself a glass of this iced herbal tea. This will satisfy the taste buds and assist your body in washing out toxins. Here are a few other gifts that the herbal world can offer you:

— In an attempt to lose weight quickly, many compulsive eaters have abused traditional pharmaceutical diuretics. As a result, the body may have difficulty releasing excess water on its own. If salty snacks have been a binge food of choice, water retention may also be an issue. **Corn silk** is a natural herbal diuretic. In China, the silk of the corn (the light yellow strands of silky material wrapped around the corn on the cob) has a long history of use as a natural diuretic. To relieve excessive water retention, use as a tea 3–4 times per day. Other useful herbal teas with diuretic properties are **dandelion** and **parsley.**

— When one consumes a great deal of processed food, constipation can be a problem. **Yellow dock,** an herb that thrives on roadsides, ditches, and even in dumps, is an **aperient.** Aperients work to assist the bowel by gently stimulating the digestive system. When treating constipation, be sure to use the root of the yellow dock herb. Drink this herbal tea preparation three times a day. If you're in need of a stronger laxative, **licorice root,** used medicinally in Europe for thousands of years; and **dandelion root,** one of my favorite herbs, both have mild laxative properties. All of these herbs can be found in teabag form at your local health food store. Be sure to use as directed.

(**Note:** If licorice is overused, it can elevate the blood pressure. Do not use this herb if you have high blood pressure. It's also recommended that this herb not be used for more than seven days in a row.)

— Here are three more herbs to consider. **Fenugreek** is an herb with an interesting history. Used as a food by the Greeks and Romans, the ancient Egyptians decided it was a necessary ingredient in embalming fluid. For our purposes, it's important to know that fenugreek can assist in dissolving fat in the liver. Buy in capsule form at a health food store, and take as directed on the label.

Fennel was used in the Middle Ages to keep the evil spirits away. The seeds were regularly stuffed into keyholes in doors to keep the ghosts out. For the individual healing from compulsive eating, fennel can be used as a natural appetite suppressant. Used in tea form, not only will this herb reduce pangs of hunger, but it will remove fat from the intestinal tract.

In medieval Europe, **hawthorn** was often associated with witches and witchcraft. It was believed that witches could turn themselves into a hawthorn tree at will. For our purposes, we can use this herb to burn off excessive calories, rid the body of excessive water and salt, strengthen the heart muscles, increase the flow of oxygen and blood to the heart, and lower cholesterol levels. Steep a tea bag of hawthorn berries in one cup of boiling water for 20 minutes, and drink this old witch's brew three times a day.

For complete healing from compulsive eating to take place, you must be willing to take complete responsibility for every area of your life. Once this commitment to the self is made, there really will be light at the end of the tunnel.

Sherry was in the lunchroom looking for Gary. They had spent the morning swimming with tropical fish in the blue-green waters of the Caribbean. Sherry was starving. As she got into the buffet line, she saw an overweight man walking away with six slices of key lime pie. *There goes a heart attack waiting to happen,* she thought. Moving up the line, she caught sight of her husband, Gary. Looking at his plate, she noticed that it was piled high with nothing but iceberg lettuce. Leaving the line, she made her way to him and asked, "What are you up to now? That isn't enough for a meal!"

As he put his plate down on the table in front of him he replied, "We will be home tomorrow. It's time to start dieting."

Sherry took his plate from him. Startled, Gary asked, "Hey! What are you doing? Give me back my rabbit food. I'm hungry!"

Sitting down next to him, Sherry questioned, "Has dieting *ever* worked for us? No. You become an irritable bear, I'm miserable, and once we quit the rabbit food, the pounds pile back on. It's time for us to do something different. No more of this quick-weight-loss, yo-yo stuff, okay?"

With this, Gary pushed the lettuce away and replied, "Okay. *Now* what do you have in mind?"

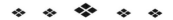

Chapter fifteen

ANOREXIA: A SLOW DEATH

All the windows in the bright yellow "house on stilts" were open. The cool, moist Gulf Coast breeze gently moved through the kitchen. Looking out at the blue ocean, Amy thought, *This year's Christmas Boat Parade is going to be a blast!* The annual parade was scheduled to take place later on that evening. She could already see some of the colorfully lit boats lined up along the docks. Turning to the stove, Amy noticed that the water for the "Cajun boil" was ready. The scent of allspice, bay leaves, red pepper, lemon, and garlic began to assault her nostrils.

Standing over the stove was her mother, Tammy, who was also looking forward to the parade. She had invited her sister, Anna, to join them. As Amy rinsed off the green beans, she asked, "When will Aunt Anna be here, Mom?"

Tammy had just dumped a bunch of fresh shrimp into the Cajun boil. Wiping her hands on her apron, she turned to her daughter and replied, "Your aunt should be here anytime." Amy put the green beans by the stove. After the shrimp and potatoes had been boiled, it would be time to add the corn and green beans.

"Mom, I need to ask you something, and it's kind of important," Amy said. "Have you ever noticed that Aunt Anna is really skinny? Even a little anorexic?"

Turning to hug her daughter, Tammy sighed and answered, "Yes, honey, your aunt *is* anorexic, and I'm really very worried about her."

Suddenly, the front door opened and slammed. "Hello? Where is everybody, and what smells so good?" Anna then cried out, "I'm starved!" As her sister walked into the kitchen, Tammy's heart sank. Anna appeared to be thinner than ever. She seemed to be lost in her clothes.

Anorexia nervosa can be an extremely frightening disease, affecting not only one out of every 250 women in our culture, but a growing number of men as well. This self-induced form of starvation is very difficult to treat as well and is affecting more and more people in our culture who are obsessed with thinness. No matter how underweight an anorexic might be, those suffering from this disorder see themselves as overweight.

For years, this disorder has been looked upon as a psychological issue that can be resolved with forced feedings, talk therapy, and traditional psychiatric medications. This method rarely works because it doesn't address the health of the whole person. The illness is also very misunderstood. Anorexia is actually a very creative survival skill. For healing to begin, it must be understood that this coping tool initially originated in order to physically, emotionally, and spiritually buffer the affected individual from the realities of life. When looking at the illness from this perspective, it becomes clear why a holistic approach to healing is essential.

The Psychology of Anorexia

When an anorexic doesn't eat, this perpetuates the illness. Electrolyte imbalances, a consequence of potassium and sodium depletion, will dramatically affect the thinking process. The mood is changed, and an "anorexic high" is induced. If laxatives are being used, this will also drain potassium levels. Low potassium levels can cause death.

(**Note:** When one suffering from this condition is physically at death's door, immediate measures must be taken before psychological issues can be instituted, such as rehydration, replacement of electrolytes, and perhaps hospitalization. Once the physical health of the individual has been somewhat improved, the thinking process will return, and the following measures can be taken.)

— **Education.** Education is the key that unlocks the door leading to eventual health. If you have concerns about your weight and others have told you that they think you're too thin, investigate the many symptoms of this disease. There are numerous books on this topic. I have written two books on food disorders, *Eat Like a Lady: A Guide to Recovery from Bulimia,* and *Am I Hungry or Am I Hurting?* These can be found at your local library.

If you've questioned yourself about the low weight of a loved one, ask other family members if they have similar concerns. Then, using the following categories, take a look at the *consequences* to weight loss:

- Tally up the amount of money spent on other physical illnesses. Anorexia often affects the menstrual cycle, energy levels, and blood pressure (which is often too low). It can bring about the onset of osteoporosis and can also lead to difficulty healing from wounds. It can also cause muscle spasms; heart palpitations; and hair, skin, nail, and dental problems.

- Examine the amount of money spent on well-meaning, but often unaware, mental health-care providers, psychologists, psychiatrists, and counselors. Many helping professionals have difficulty identifying, let alone treating, this disease.

- List the amount of time spent on weight obsession, looking in the mirror, feeling fat, trying new diets, exercising, obsessing on food and the amount of food eaten; weighing oneself, or just feeling blue about the physical body.

- Look at how this obsession has interfered with relationships, jobs, schooling, goals, hobbies, and family gatherings. If life rotates around the illness, there's no room for spirituality.

Categorically listing the many consequences of this illness can be a real eye-opener.

— It's important to determine why this creative **core survival skill** was developed. The following visualization will help:

Close your eyes and relax. Visualize your obsession to be thin. Give it physical form with a personality. Maybe this obsession will look like a runway model or perfectly shaped physical body. Ask this vision how old it is. What is the very first number that pops into your head? Once you have a number, visualize yourself at this age. For instance, if the first number you think of is 12, visualize yourself at that age. Ask this young version of you why it thinks it is fat. If there's no response, visualize a playground full of kids. Ask the group, "Who thinks they're fat?" Once you've identified individuals in the group who see themselves as overweight, understand that this person is you. After identifying this image, ask, "Why do you think you're fat?" Listen carefully for the answer. The obsession with weight usually begins in childhood or adolescence. When life feels out of control, the young person learns that the one thing he or she can control is what is eaten.

Finally, ask this person, "How is life? What upsets you? Who makes you angry, sad, or scared?" After listening to all that is said, write down what you've learned. If this exercise is impossible to do, seek out the assistance of a therapist, spiritual advisor, or holistic helping professional.

— **Unresolved issues.** As long as one is focused on body weight, this distances the person from dealing with unresolved life issues of the present and past. Painful problems with school, friends, parents, marriage, divorce, and more can be buried beneath the obsession of anorexia. Previous difficulties with work, alcohol, drugs, food, or sexually dysfunctional caregivers will give rise to this illness. Living with caregivers who have unresolved traumas of their own can perpetuate this affliction in children. Also, the death or loss of a loved one often provides fertile ground for the this affliction. The painful emotions related to unresolved physical, emotional, or sexual trauma can also be held at bay by self-starvation, and these issues should never be ignored.

Remember, this creative survival skill alters mood and is effective in defending against emotional pain. Exploring just what that hurt might be is essential for healing to begin. This process of exploration often proves to be difficult. If this is the case, find a therapist who not only understands food addictions, but who uses a holistic approach to treatment.

Lifestyle Remedies for Coping with Anorexia

Initial lifestyle changes involve family members because they tend to be a big part of the problem. If the family develops new, healthy coping skills for dealing with anorexic behavior, the health of the sufferer will begin to improve.

— At the onset of the illness, most anorexics tend to have normal feelings of hunger. Eventually, they learn to ignore them. Remember, anorexia is about control. The statement, "I'm just not hungry" can hook family members into devoting massive amounts of time to the weight and food habits of an extremely thin loved one. Interestingly, individuals who suffer from this condition tend to be obsessed with recipes, vitamins, and the feeding of pets, and will even prepare elaborate meals. Sadly, when it's time to eat the meal, the cook in this case will take very little food for her- or himself, confusing friends and family members. Tempers can flare when family members state, "You need to eat." The anorexic often feels that he or she is being controlled (there's that word again), and the response usually is, "I'm not hungry. You're just jealous because I'm thin," or "I just don't eat as much as you do."

After such a battle, family members may find themselves believing the excuses an anorexic loved one has offered. Comments fueling the denial of this disorder may include, "Oh, honey, I'm sorry. You're not too thin," or "Yes, Uncle Gene is just jealous. You know how he likes to eat," or "Well, maybe you're naturally slim and really do need less food than the rest of us," or "How can that doctor say your blood pressure is related to your weight?"

Adapting a lifestyle that involves **learning not to rescue or react** to anorexic behavior is extremely important. This new behavior promotes health in the family and encourages the affected friend or family member to begin taking responsibility for him- or herself.

— **Personal responsibility.** It's important to know that the fear of being fat can often be tied to apprehension about growing up. If you're anorexic, it's imperative that you recognize that only *you* can heal yourself from this ailment. Taking responsibility for yourself is a must, but it can be done with baby steps.

A realistic goal for self-healing involves implementing some kind of daily eating pattern. At this point, quality and quantity are not important. Setting up a habit of eating and drinking a little something on a regular basis will hopefully lay the groundwork for a healthy eating plan. (Nutritional supplements will play a major role in establishing physical health.) If you want to eat a slice of pizza for breakfast, raw cabbage for lunch, and an egg for dinner, that's great. The goal is to eat a bit of food, three times a day. An intake of 4–8 oz. of water, herbal tea, and fresh juice, eight times a day, is another short-term lifestyle goal to shoot for. After these two objectives have been consistently met for several months, then it will be time to focus more on consuming a complete meal.

— Identifying a **particular time of day** when it feels most comfortable to eat is the next step. At this time, a small meal will be eaten. Once again, quantity isn't important, but quality is. A meal consisting of one protein dish, a starch, and a vegetable should be prepared. What is put on your plate needs to be *your* decision. At least one bite of each dish should be taken. Because the fear of getting fat can kick in at this time, it might be necessary to write about feelings immediately after eating. Remember, the fear of getting fat distances you from your emotions. Ingesting food and filling the stomach can produce an out-of-control feeling, as well as a host of emotions. If necessary, after eating, attendance at a support group such as the American

Anorexia/Bulimia Association, Overeaters Anonymous, or Adult Children of Alcoholics can aid in processing the feelings that arise at this time.

— Develop **creativity** and **spirituality.** Spirituality and creativity must be explored. Getting together with other individuals who have had to confront difficult life issues can be a spiritual experience. Joining with those in support groups, meditation classes, therapy groups, self-help organizations, or church groups can break down the sense of uniqueness and isolation. Looking into yoga, painting, guitar playing, dancing, singing, cooking, sculpting, theater work, writing, piano playing, or any other creative activity also encourages spiritual development. Finding a creative activity that is enjoyable can aid in increasing self-esteem. As a positive sense of self develops, intimate relationships are not as frightening. When intimate friendships increase, spirituality can begin to blossom.

Recognizing that this illness does not define you will free you to investigate those areas of your life that you've neglected. Under the guise of an anorexic identity, there can be an artist, writer, lover, teacher, musician, poet, healer, parent, and beautiful person. Discovering just who the self is does involve risk, and self-discovery can initially be very frightening. Is it worth it? Yes.

Spirituality also begins when one learns how to nurture the body, mind, and soul. For those of us who are anorexic, it's important to know that the first step in nurturing the self has to begin with learning how to nurture the body.

Nutritional and Herbal Support for Healing the Body

Because the nutritional state of the individual plagued with anorexia is so deficient, immediate nonthreatening steps must be taken to remedy this problem. If an individual is near death due to self-starvation, tube feeding to reestablish stability may be necessary. Focus should then be placed on the following nutritional steps, in order of presentation. This program will not immediately put weight on an underweight individual. What it *will* do is begin replacing nutritionally deficient states within the physical body with those vitamins and minerals necessary to begin the healing process.

— **Look at Appendix II.** It's extremely important that these recommendations for nutritional supplementation be followed. When using supplements, purchase those that are easily absorbed by the system. Ask a health food store clerk which brand of supplements can be gently digested. Along with the vitamin supplements recommended in Appendix II, the following supplementation is advised. (If the anorexic condition is severe, use multivitamin and mineral supplements in spray form. These can be found at your local health food store.)

- **Natural beta carotene:** 25,000 IU per day
- **Vitamin A:** 10,000 IU per day
- **Calcium:** 1,500 mg per day in two doses
- **Magnesium:** 1,000 mg per day in two doses
- **Potassium:** 99 mg per day
- **Selenium:** 200 mcg per day
- **Zinc:** 80 mg per day. This particular nutrient assists individuals in regaining a healthy, normal appetite.
- **Copper:** 3 mg per day. Take this supplement separately from zinc.
- **Acidophilus:** This nutrient replaces friendly bacteria lost through vomiting or laxative abuse and should be taken as directed on the label.

- **Free-form amino acid complex:** This nutrient is needed to encourage tissue repair, lost with starvation. Take as directed on the label.

- **Vitamin B complex:** The Bs are needed to correct anemic conditions and to replace lost B vitamins. Take 100 mg three times per day.

- **Vitamin B12 injections:** 1 cc three times per week will increase the appetite, repair any damage done to the body, and will assist in preventing hair loss, common with self-starvation and illness.

- **Liver extract injections:** 2 cc three times per week will supply necessary B vitamins along with other valuable nutrients.

- **Valuable Vitamin C:** 5,000 mg daily, divided into three separate doses. This vitamin is needed to repair the immune system and the overstressed adrenal glands.

- **Floradix iron and herbs from Salus Haus:** This product is a natural source of iron and should be taken as directed on the label.

- **Brewer's yeast:** One teaspoon of this nutrient per day provides another source of balanced B vitamins.

- **Kelp:** Food from the ocean, full of essential vitamins and minerals. Take as directed on the label.

- **Proteolytic enzymes:** Take this nutritional supplement in between meals and with meals as directed on the label. It assists with digestion and aids in building tissue.

- **Vitamin D:** 600 IU per day. This particular nutrient helps the body absorb calcium and prevent bone loss.

- **Vitamin E:** 600 IU per day. This vitamin assists in healing by encouraging oxygen uptake in the body.

Vitamins are not fattening, and as a result, they're usually not threatening to an underweight individual. Although fearful of food, most anorexics tend to understand that it's necessary to improve the body's nutritional status. Transforming behavior from the obsession of not wanting to eat to obtaining optimal physical health is an essential baby step for healing.

— **Fruit and vegetable juices.** The psychological goal of initial nutritional healing is to make the food ingested feel "safe." Fresh fruit juices are not only low in calories, but are full of vitamins and minerals. Additionally, they're easy to digest and quickly absorbed. So get out that juicer and start experimenting with different fruit and veggie combinations. If needed, pick up a recipe book on juicing at a local health food store. Start out this healthy venture by having 2–3 ounces of fresh vegetable or fruit juice four times per day, and gradually increase your intake.

— A person who is phobic about gaining weight will naturally gravitate toward **diet foods.** This is perfectly fine, so long as the chosen foods are nutritious. Cooked vegetables served in their juices are extremely low in calories, very nutritious, and easy to digest. A healthy "no pressure" meal for the person healing from anorexia might be fruit and fat-free yogurt. A small portion of beans with rice is high in protein, as is a fresh salad topped off with fat-free cottage cheese and a bit of fat-free cheese. Made from soybeans, tofu is regarded as the "weird" food of the new millennium by those who aren't familiar with it. But tofu taste differs by brand, and preparation can also affect the taste greatly. Trust me—I eat it all of the time. Tofu is very low in calories and is extremely nutritious.

— **Avoid** the following high-fat, empty calorie items: white flour, white sugar, junk foods, processed foods, diet soft drinks (which interfere with calcium absorption), alcohol (which interferes with the absorption of many vitamins), and caffeine. If caffeinated beverages are being used, cut down on their consumption.

The above suggestions are just a few of the many natural options that can be utilized to begin healing from anorexia. Within the world of herbs, there are several other natural remedies that fit nicely into a holistic healing approach for anorexia.

— **Dandelion.** This herb has so many healing properties. It really is one of my favorites. Ancient herbal folklore suggests that if you blow dandelion seeds into the wind, you'll be able to send your thoughts to a loved one. Dandelion tea is very nutritious, full of vitamins A, B, C, and D. This herb is also rich in calcium. Because of its potassium content, it's useful for balancing out the electrolytes. Dandelion leaf tea is readily available in most health food stores. Serve with a touch of honey, and drink throughout the day.

— **Ginger root.** Once thought to have its origins in the Garden of Eden, this plant has been valued in Asia since the earliest of times. The spicy herb makes a wonderfully flavored tea. It also relieves nausea and improves the appetite. To increase circulation and improve digestion, drink it several times a day. It can also be used in a glycerin tincture form. Take as directed on the label.

— "I want my **peppermint** tummy tea" is a common request around my house. The smell of this herb is uplifting and stimulating. My son loves this tea served hot with a bit of honey. Peppermint will assist digestion and calm a nervous stomach.

— **St. John's wort.** Once believed to be capable of making evil spirits disappear, it's now recognized that St. John's wort contains a psychotropic constituent called hypericum. This particular constituent can assist in relieving mild depression. During the 19th century, this herb was put on the back shelf, but recently it has made a major comeback as a useful medicinal herb. St. John's wort is so popular that it can be found in tea, tinctures, and capsule form at most health food stores. Use as directed on the label.

For an individual healing from anorexia, herbal teas provide many benefits and can be of great healing value. Some herbal teas are nutritious, while others are calming. There are also many herbal teas that just taste good. Because herbal teas are calorie-free, they also provide a tasty, nonthreatening means for addressing the dehydration that often accompanies anorexia. Hibiscus, strawberry, and orange herbal tea all have a wonderful scent and naturally sweet flavor. These are my favorite herbal teas to have on ice during the summertime.

Addressing anorexia with a holistic approach takes time and courage, but it also increases the probability of total healing. Because anorexia is often difficult for family, friends—and the sufferer—to understand, it's important to recognize that identification of this problem is the first step to recovery.

After the Christmas Boat Parade, Tammy and Anna were sitting on the back porch. Tammy had just brewed up a pot of dandelion tea, and the sisters were admiring the boats in their Christmas finery. As Tammy poured her sister a cup of the steamy golden liquid, she said, "Anna, because I love you, I need to tell you something."

"What is it, Sis?" Anna asked.

Tammy took her sister's hand in hers and said, "Ever since

Mom died five years ago, I've watched you get thinner and thinner."

Suddenly pulling her hand away, Anna stood up, crossed her arms over her chest and said, "Not you, too. Dad says the same thing. I'm not too skinny."

Tammy calmly put her tea cup down and replied, "Yes, you are, and I'm not going to pretend anymore. It hurts me to watch you self-destruct in this way. You're anorexic, and you're using this behavior to alter your mood, to keep you from feeling the pain of Mom's death. I love you and want you to be happy, but your healing is up to you." Anna was furious, but Tammy continued. "If you choose to travel this path—not eat, see yourself as fat, and lose more weight—I can't stop you. But I will no longer act as if it's not happening. I'm going to go get some information on anorexia and educate myself." Tammy got up and went through the door leading to the kitchen.

Anna sat alone on the porch for about an hour. When she came back into the house, she looked at Tammy and said, "Sis, I'm scared."

Tammy embraced her sister and said, "I know."

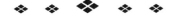

Chapter sixteen

BULIMIA: RUNNING ON EMPTY

Marsha grabbed the potato salad and made a run for the back door. As she forced the door open with her shoulder, she thought, *They will all be here in ten minutes.* Once outside in the backyard, Marsha put the salad down on the picnic table and then quickly checked the barbecue smoker. Lifting the lid, the scent of smoked albacore escaped into the air.

"The fish smells great, Mom. When do we start the hot dogs?" asked her young son, Timmy. Picking up a baseball, Timmy yelled, "Hey, Mom, think fast." He tossed the ball to his mother. Marsha barely caught the ball, and then laughed. She really was looking forward to seeing the whole family.

While taking the baked potatoes out of the oven, Marsha heard the doorbell ring. All of the relatives had shown up at once, and everyone crowded into the living room. The relatives greeted one another with hugging, talking, teasing, and the cheek-pinching of children. As Marsha made her way through the warm embraces of her parents, grandparents, aunts, and uncles, she saw her cousin Jack come through the door. Her once-joyous mood quickly evaporated. It had been 20 years since she had laid eyes on this cousin, and seeing him brought the pain of the past to the present. *If he touches me*, she thought, *I don't know what I'll do.*

After everyone had eaten, Marsha went into the kitchen to get the chocolate pies she had made for dessert. Placing the desserts on a serving tray, she then returned to the party in the backyard. Chocolate pie was something she usually avoided, but this afternoon she decided not to just have one piece, but four. As she ate, she couldn't even taste the rich chocolate or enjoy the sweet whipped topping. After eating her dessert, Marsha began collecting and scraping dishes. While doing so, she quickly ate several cold hot dogs. Suddenly, Jack walked through the kitchen door. He was getting another beer, and as he closed the refrigerator, he asked, "Marsha, how about a hug? You aren't trying to avoid me, are you?"

Seeing him brought back the terror of a night two decades ago. It was as if she could feel him molesting her all over again. As he made his way toward her, she said, "Excuse me," and headed straight for the bathroom. Once the bathroom door was locked, Marsha found herself throwing up not only her dinner, but the hot dogs and four pieces of chocolate pie.

The severe illness bulimia nervosa affects a large number of people today. With this condition, there's a compulsion to binge on large quantities of food. When compulsively eating, the mind is altered with the food. Numb with the intake of often highly processed, white flour, white sugary, salty, high-fat food, current life difficulties or past traumas can be momentarily repressed. The binge behavior is then followed by a strong compulsion to purge the body of either the food or the calories associated with it. Purging behavior can consist of vomiting, laxative abuse, excessive use of enemas, abuse of diuretics, ingesting an inordinate amount of fiber foods, or extreme exercise regimens. After losing control with bingeing, the purge provides a false sense of control. The purge behavior is also mind-altering.

This illness can take a toll on the human body. With constant purging, dehydration can be a real problem, creating an imbalance in the electrolytes. This disruption can lead to heart failure. With vomiting, the stomach acid destroys teeth, dissolving the protective enamel, often turning them gray. Other physical consequences of this affliction include internal bleeding, ulcers, erratic heartbeat, kidney damage, hypoglycemia, low blood pressure, irregular menstrual cycles, or a ruptured stomach. Traditional treatment typically involves antidepressants and "talk" therapy. Sadly, with this method, relapse is common. In utilizing a more holistic approach, it's understood that bulimia affects the whole person. Let's begin this process of healing by exploring the psychology behind the condition.

The Psychology of Bulimia

— **The food journal is a must.** Why is the need to binge and then purge so strong? The food journal is essential to answering this question. Bingeing and purging patterns are always preceded by some life experience that has induced strong emotions. In your journal, food ingested for the day needs to be listed, along with bouts of purging. Quantity of food eaten also needs to be inventoried. Honesty is a must, because the quantity of food ingested tends to increase with stress. Examining the stresses that were in your life 24 to 48 hours before a binge or purge began will assist you in grasping just how this survival skill has been working for you. Seeing the behavior as a mood-altering protective mechanism will clearly demonstrate that the bulimia is a coping mechanism. Write in the food journal for two weeks.

— Looking at **core issues.** As mentioned earlier, bulimia originates for a reason. Some individuals come from families where alcoholism, drug addiction, physical violence, or sexual abuse was prevalent. For others, there's a sense of never feeling "good enough," believing life's problems will disappear if only the physical body were more attractive or perfect. These core issues are tough to address. As a result, it's not uncommon for the desire to binge and purge to increase during the initial phases of psychological healing. At this time, it's important to understand that the goal of healing is to recognize how the behavior is tied to core issues, and that it's necessary to begin limiting the number of binge-purge episodes you have. With the help of a therapist, support group, spiritual advisor, or alternative health-care provider, the issues that perpetuate bulimia can be resolved. Use the following visualization to begin identifying your core issues.

Close your eyes, and visualize yourself at the time you first binged and purged. Ask this image of yourself what the need was to do this. Question why the body seems to be reviled. Listen to what is said. Then inquire, "Who else hates your body?" Notice how the image responds to this particular question. Now ask, "Are you lovable?" What is the reaction to this question?

(**Note:** If the image disappears, this is often related to fear of the question being asked. Open your eyes and write about your experience. Then list the major events in your life that have made you feel extremely sad or angry. If you still have strong emotions about these situations, these are your unresolved core issues. This is your unfinished business, and you need to take time to heal.)

—**Self-forgiveness.** Most bulimics feel a great deal of shame about their bingeing and purging behavior. "If others knew what I did behind the locked bathroom door, they would hate me," is what I often hear from bulimics. Bulimia is a secretive illness. For this reason, it's important to find one person to share this behavior with. The person you discuss your bulimia with needs to be nonjudgmental, accepting, and supportive. Acceptance from another will encourage you to forgive yourself. Also, use the following meditation to facilitate self-forgiveness.

Visualize the bulimia, and give it a form you can focus on. This might be massive amounts of unhealthy food or any other image that fits for you. Initially, you will feel a great deal of repulsion for this image. Imagine screaming at the bulimia, "I hate you!" If you need to, beat on a pillow while you visualize pounding on the bulimia. Once the rage has been expressed, it's not uncommon for this emotion to be replaced with a sense of sadness, which can be very strong. You may feel grief about having had to destroy the health of your body to survive the stresses and traumas of life. As time goes on, you will begin to acknowledge the bulimia as a survival skill. Your sadness will eventually move to a sense of appreciation. Once you see this, you will be able to forgive yourself for being bulimic.

— **Your body is not the enemy.** Many bulimics use the media as a gauge for how the human body should look, not understanding that this is fantasy. To create the illusion of perfection, the photographs of most celebrities have been touched up. Numerous models have risked their health to obtain a rail-thin look through anorexia, bulimia, extreme diets, or excessive plastic surgery. In the real world, the human body comes in all shapes and sizes. Activities such as dance, yoga, meditation, message therapy, or gazing at yourself in a full-length mirror can begin to connect you with your body in a healthy manner. I have yet to see a "perfect" body in a yoga class consisting of real, everyday people. Learning to love and appreciate one's body takes time, but it's a start.

Essential Lifestyle Changes for Recovering from Bulimia

On the outside, most bulimics appear confident and self-assured, but behind closed doors they're steeped in low self-esteem and insecurity. Lifestyle changes must involve breaking free from the enclosed secret prison that this illness often creates.

— **Support groups** specifically for bulimia or food addictions can be very shame-reducing. Sitting in a room with others who are wrestling with similar difficulties tends to remove that sense of "I'm the only one and I'm such a freak," and replaces it with, "Hey, they know exactly how I feel!" Therapy sessions, 12-step meetings, women's and men's groups, or any type of intimate setting can promote safe, honest, open sharing, and acceptance of the self.

— **Balanced exercise.** B-A-L-A-N-C-E. Before going any further, it's very important to note that some bulimics have used excessive exercise as a method of purging calories. If you've done this, it's important for you to understand that a healthy exercise program is balanced, not extreme. Used properly, a healthy exercise program can reap many positive rewards. Once purging behavior ceases, it isn't uncommon for a bulimic to gain a few extra pounds. (I know, some of you are freaking out as you read this. Take a deep breath and read on.) The condition is temporary, and a healthy exercise program can reduce your anxiety. A balanced program of exercise, consisting of no less than 30 minutes per day and no more than an hour per day, contributes to a greater sense of well-being. Having a variety of activities to choose from, such as walking, swimming, kayaking, ice skating, rowing, dancing, weight lifting, hiking, skiing, wind surfing, and walking the dog can make exercise a very important and enjoyable part of recovery.

— **Prayer and meditation.** When you're feeling overwhelmed by the desire to binge or purge, prayer can be of great assistance. Asking one's concept of God or a Higher Power to provide the strength necessary to keep from acting-out can help keep a binge/purge cycle at bay. Developing a spirituality for today may involve removing destructive or frightening God concepts from youth. In situations such as this, assistance from a helping professional can be a blessing. Such a helper will encourage you to develop your own concept of a loving God or a higher spiritual principle.

Nutritional and Herbal Support for Healing the Body

Like the compulsive eater, those suffering from bulimia can be very malnourished. Bingeing on high-fat, sugary, over-processed foods void of any nutritional value, and then purging with vomiting, starves the body. Laxative abuse washes much-needed sodium and potassium from the system. Both laxative abuse and vomiting create electrolyte imbalances and dehydration. Vitamin and mineral deficiencies, along with electrolyte disparity, can lead to hair loss, yellow skin, premature wrinkles, bad breath, depression, fatigue, dizziness, muscle weakness, and degenerative diseases. Nutritional issues must be addressed if psychological difficulties are to be successfully resolved.

— **Return to the food journal** to determine exactly what your diet consists of. When using the food journal with bulimics, I have noticed that most binge foods consist of cakes, cookies, candy, ice cream, chips, dips, gravies, heavy sauces, pizza, doughnuts, cheesy macaroni, breads with loads of jam or butter, and peanut butter. Foods not thrown up or purged in other ways tend to be skimpy salads or diet-type foods. Few of these foods provide complete nutrition for health. Some bulimics throw up anything ingested, and this can produce extreme malnutrition. To top this off, caffeine-laced diet sodas tend to be the drink of choice. Caffeine also dehydrates and robs the body of valuable nutrients. The high phosphorus content found in diet sodas can interfere with calcium absorption. Lack of calcium leads to weak teeth and bones. Reviewing the food journal will give you a great deal of information about your nutritional state.

— **Education.** Yes, it's essential to begin exploring what a healthy diet consists of. Remember, don't expect instant success. *Progress* is the word. Forget perfection. Perfection is part of the problem. After years of bulimic behavior, developing a nutritionally sound diet will take time. Begin this phase of healing by eating one nutritionally sound meal per day. Have this meal at a time (according to the food journal) when binge/purge behavior is least likely to occur. This meal can be the foundation for building a list of healthy, non-binge-type foods.

For this particular meal, certain foods should be avoided. Avoid all fast foods, fried foods, processed foods, red meat, refined sugar, saturated fats, and dairy products, except for unsweetened yogurt and skim milk. The foods making up this meal must be as fresh as possible and not include white-flour products. Alcohol should also be avoided. This first consistent healthy daily meal cannot include any of the foods you regularly binge on. That means that if tofu or oat bran muffins are past binge foods, they need to be avoided.

Nutritious foods for this meal should be high in fiber, with many raw and cooked vegetables, fruits, legumes, grains, a few nuts, and seeds. For hydration of the dehydrated bulimic condition, herbal teas and fresh vegetable juices also need to be included in the meal. If you're a meat eater, small amounts of broiled, baked, grilled, or stir-fried skinless chicken, turkey, or fish can be included in this meal.

Be sure to experiment with the above food groups. Find recipes that suit your taste buds. Once you've been able to eat, without purging, one daily meal for six months, then begin this process again with a second nutritious meal for the day. Know that during this initial six-month period, you may periodically binge and purge. The only goal you need to have at this time is to not purge this one nutritious meal. As you develop more healthy life skills for addressing daily stress, intense emotion, and past trauma, the desire to binge and purge will begin to diminish. Since the process of developing a healthy nutritional food plan will take time, nutritional supplements will be absolutely necessary.

— Begin this step by referring to the **Supplement for Health Program** found in Appendix II. While healing from bulimia, it's suggested that the multivitamin and mineral complex suggested in this Appendix be taken with meals for better absorption. In the book *Prescriptions for Nutritional Healing,* the following additional nutritional supplements are listed specifically for bulimia. Take these, along with those suggested in the **Supplement for Health Program.**

- **Vitamin A**—15,000 IU total per day (unless pregnant; if pregnant, only 10,000 IU per day)
- **Natural beta carotene**—25,000 IU total per day

(**Note:** Hopefully, a good multivitamin will contain the above two nutrients. Do not use a sustained formula, because these two nutrients tend to pass through the intestinal tract rather quickly, thus interfering with absorption ability.)

- **Selenium**—This nutrient is a vital antioxidant that helps protect the immune system by preventing the formation of damaging free radicals. Take as directed on the label.

- **Zinc**—Don't forget the zinc: 50–100 mg per day. This mineral assists in protein metabolism and provides you with a sense of taste. Zinc deficiency is very common in bulimics.

(**Note:** Do not exceed a total of 100 mg per day. Check the zinc content in your multivitamin and mineral supplement before adding this supplement to your daily program.)

- **Copper**—3 mg per day. This particular mineral is needed to balance out zinc. Do not take zinc with copper. If the multivitamin and mineral supplement contains zinc, take the copper supplement later.

- **Acidophilus**—Take as directed on the label. This nutrient promotes healthy intestinal bacteria in the gastrointestinal system, and it assists in protecting the liver.

- **Calcium**—1,500 mg nightly. This mineral calms the nervous system and replenishes the body with needed calcium.

- **Magnesium**—750 mg nightly. Don't forget to take your magnesium with your calcium supplement. Magnesium assists with calcium absorption, and it relaxes smooth muscles.

- **Free-form amino acid complex**—Take as directed on the label. This product is helpful in counteracting the serious protein deficiency found with bulimia.

- **Vitamin B complex**—100 mg per day. This is necessary for proper cellular function.

- **Vitamin B12 injections**—1 cc three times per week from a qualified health-care provider. This nutrient is needed to assist in digestion and for the assimilation of nutrients, including iron.
- **Liver extract supplements** (if not a vegetarian)— Take as directed on the label. This is a good source of not only B vitamins, but other nutrients as well.
- **Vitamin C**—No, don't forget the C. Take 5,000 mg per day divided into two to three doses. Be sure the vitamin is buffered C. This nutrient is not only necessary for all glandular and cellular function, but it also assists in improving immunity.

Before a healthy nutritional food program has been totally implemented, these nutritional supplements will help you heal your body, enhance your immune system, and gain strength. This, in turn, will clear your mind and thinking processes. As you begin to feel better emotionally and physically, you will feel more at ease with your meal plan. In turn, you will be able to resolve those psychological core issues that originally set up this illness.

Now it's time to see what the herb world has for your healing journey. In this first section on herbs, we will be looking at those remedies that are useful for emotional upset.

(**A note of caution:** Herbs will interact with prescription medications. If you're currently taking traditional psychotropic medications or other mood-altering prescription drugs, it's strongly suggested that you not use the following herbs.)

— Many bulimics suffer from anxiety attacks and depression. The world of herbs has several solutions. In medieval Europe, **St. John's wort** flowers were considered to have powerful magic abilities. This was thought to be especially true during the summer solstice. Hypericum, the red-colored oil contained within the yellow-flowering tops of this plant, has antidepressant qualities. Because most bulimics suffer from depression, St. John's wort can aid in elevating the mood. Drink this herb in tea form three times a day.

(**Note:** This herb can cause sensitivity to sunlight. Use sunscreen if you go outside.)

— **Vervain** was very popular with the Druids. The ancient spiritual leaders used this herb to sweep sacred spaces for rituals and as a charm against curses and bad luck. Vervain will relax the entire nervous system and is a great remedy for stress or tension. Use as directed in an alcohol-free tincture or tea.

— **Skullcap** was a favorite medicinal herb for the Cherokee Indians. Like vervain, it, too, is very effective for reducing anxiety. When feeling overwhelmed, instead of grabbing a cup of coffee or diet soda, brew up a cup of skullcap tea. Skullcap tea can be taken three times a day, or as needed. I keep this herb in tea form at my office and home.

— Let's take a look at **alfalfa,** an herb that can aid the body in absorbing nutrients. No, it's not just for cows. The American Indians used alfalfa as a food source. This herb contains the following nutrients: alpha-carotene; beta-carotene; B-complex vitamins; calcium; chlorophyll; copper; essential amino acids; iron; magnesium; phosphorus; potassium; protein; sodium sulfur; sulfur; zinc; and vitamins A, C, D, E, and K. For the malnourished body, alfalfa is loaded with goodies. Use in tea or tablet form as directed on the label.

(**Note:** Do not use alfalfa if you're taking a traditional pharmaceutical blood anticoagulation.)

— One of the nine sacred herbs of the Anglo-Saxons is **fennel.** This herb is very restorative and is also a natural appetite suppressant. Use as directed in tea or capsule form. **Nettles** were very popular in the 17th century. In the British countryside, the herb was even used in the production of beer. Full of nutrients, nettle tea can be taken several times a day.

As mentioned earlier, when recovering from bulimia, dehydration must be remedied. Drinking flavorful herbal teas, hot or iced, can make this a pleasurable part of the healing process. Lemon balm tea was taken regularly by the 13th-century prince, Llewellyn of Glamorgan, and he supposedly lived to be 108 years old. Blackberry tea is very high in Vitamin C and is especially tasty when served iced, with sliced strawberries. Elder flower tea was once planted on the graves of the Welsh. If the flower blossomed, the departed soul was believed to be happy in the land of Tir-nan-og, a sort of Welsh heaven. Serve this tea hot on a cold day with a slice of orange or lemon rind. At grocery and health food stores, there are many packaged herbal teas. Mixing various herbal teas can produce some extremely interesting flavors and colors. Having a pitcher of herbal tea available at all times will remind you to drink up and hydrate your body.

If bulimia is holding you hostage, it's imperative that you begin to break free. A life rotating around this addiction is a waste. Holistic recovery takes a great deal of patience, dedication, and time. If you truly want to heal and are willing to look at your physical, emotional, and nutritional needs—and your lifestyle—you can escape the prison of this ailment. As you begin your journey toward freedom, be kind to yourself.

After she purged, Marsha felt just awful. For months, everything had been going so well. As she rinsed her face with cold water, she thought, *He abused me. Why do I continue to abuse me? It wasn't my fault. He just isn't worth this self-abuse.* After drying her face and hands, Marsha made her way to her bedroom to telephone one of her friends. "I really do need some support right now, and I'm going to take the time to get it because I'm worth it," she vowed.

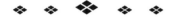

PART VII

The Balanced Woman

❧ ❧ ❧ ❧

Chapter seventeen

PREMENSTRUAL SYNDROME: AN OPPORTUNITY TO HEAL

Janie noticed that there wasn't any dishwashing soap, so she grabbed some laundry detergent, dumped a small amount in the dishwasher, closed it, and then switched the machine on. "There. That's done. Now I can go get ready for my big date." While drying her hands on a dishrag, she became dreamy eyed as she visualized her six-foot-tall, brown-eyed boyfriend. Once in her room, makeup, clothes, electric curlers, and nail polish were all that she could think of.

"Oh, my God! What on earth is happening?" yelled her mother, Norma, from the kitchen.. The dishwasher was chugging along, but with each chug, it was spewing out soap suds, *lots* of soap suds. The kitchen floor was covered with fluffy, white bubbles. Norma's face turned red as a beet as she cried out, "Janie, get down here right now." Norma then sank to the floor and burst into tears.

Waving her just-painted green fingernails in the air, Janie appeared at the kitchen doorway. "Geez, what a mess. Let me help," she said as she grabbed a towel and began sopping up the soap. "We were out of dishwashing detergent, so I dumped a bit of laundry soap into the dishwasher. I didn't know it would do this!" Without warning, Norma grabbed the dish towel from her daughter and screeched, "You never think of anybody else except yourself! You're such a selfish child, worrying only about your hair and nails."

Upon hearing his wife's escalating rage, Norma's husband, Marvin, came into the kitchen and said, "Norma, it was just a simple mistake. You're getting too worked up over this." With tears rolling down her face, Norma ran to her bedroom, slammed the door, and threw herself on her bed. As she sobbed into her pillow, she asked herself, "What on earth did I just do?"

For years, premenstrual syndrome (PMS) has been horribly misunderstood. In centuries gone by, women suffering from PMS were said to be histrionic or neurotic. Even today, after hearing complaints related to this condition, many medical doctors will shake their heads and give suffering women the name of a psychiatrist. The psychiatrist will then prescribe a variety of tranquilizers, strong diuretics, and antidepressants, never questioning the woman's stress level, lifestyle, or diet.

According to experts who understand PMS, this condition, also known as congestive dysmenorrhea, affects 90 percent of all women at one time or another in their lives. One to two weeks before the onset of the menstrual cycle, certain hormonal changes can create dramatic effects on the female body. For some women, the symptoms are very minor, while for others, PMS disrupts their family life, career, and physical health. Let's look at just a few of the 150 symptoms related to this condition.

For many women, irritation and depression can feel debilitating. As the mood swings from depression to hypersensitivity to even rage, the emotions seem overwhelming. Anxiety, insomnia, sudden outbursts, crying jags, mental confusion, forgetfulness, and nervousness are also prevalent. Experts tell us that this sudden change in mood is a result of hormonal imbalances. Estrogen levels can be very high, while progesterone is too low, or progesterone is flowing and estrogen has taken a nosedive. Any imbalance in the female sex hormones can create emotional chaos for a woman. Sugar cravings can also strike during PMS. During this time, the desire for chocolates or sweets can be maddening for women, especially if they're trying to watch their weight. For some, hypoglycemic symptoms of dizziness, heart palpitations, and low energy can also occur. Blame the hormone-like compounds called prostaglandins for these little pleasures. Excessive aldosterone, another hormone, is responsible for the fluid retention that often takes place one to two weeks before the menstrual cycle begins. Some women gain as much as five pounds in water weight and suffer from bloated abdomens, fingers, sore breasts, and general tenderness.

By now you might be saying, "The joys of being a woman. I guess I'm doomed to tolerate two weeks of torture every month until I hit menopause." Well, we are *not* powerless over PMS. If you follow a holistic treatment program for this condition, you can learn how to manage your hormones.

Understanding the Psychology of PMS

— **Talk to Mom.** Women tend to have menstrual cycles, pregnancies, and menopause experiences that are similar to those of their mothers. Talking to the older women in our families can be very normalizing. Get together with your mother, grandmother, or aunt for a PMS brain-picking session. Ask these woman to describe their experiences with their menstrual cycles.

— **Feel the feelings. It's not a sin.** The intense feelings that accompany PMS should never be suppressed. Instead, PMS days should be used to process such sensitivities. Because PMS creates a state of hypersensitivity, those emotions we easily disregarded several days ago now seem to hit us like a tidal wave. PMS makes it more difficult to ignore strong feelings that not only have been there all along, but may have been building for some time. Learning how to properly express these emotions is the key to using PMS for healing and resolving old problems. When overwhelming feelings hit, take time to write out what's bothering you. Is it low self-esteem, loss, feeling unappreciated, old unfinished business such as marital problems, financial woes, sexual issues, or communication difficulties in one of your relationships? Could it be unresolved childhood issues or difficulty with your kids? If you need help resolving these issues, ask for it.

— **Examine your anger.** "Pretty is as pretty does." How often I heard this statement from my blue-haired grandmother. As a child, I never learned how to have healthy anger, but a good case of PMS eventually forced me to examine this strong emotion. A couple of decades ago, just days before my menstrual cycle, it was not uncommon for me to erupt like a volcano. After such eruptions, I would feel just awful. Then I would beg forgiveness from anyone who had been exposed to my volatile mood, never examining what I was actually angry about. Learning how to express anger as it arises assists us in not having to blow a fuse at inappropriate times.

Make a list of all of your disappointments over the last several months, and then ask yourself, "What did I do with my anger?" Anger can surface as regret, depression, irritation, frustration, compulsive behavior, migraine headaches, or self-destructive acting-out. Getting physical by hitting tennis or golf balls, or by stomping on aluminum soda cans in the garage, can help us to discharge anger appropriately.

— **Cry if you need to.** Periodically feeling blue is perfectly normal. Loss, misunderstandings, and life's calamities will leave us feeling sad at one time or another. During PMS, sadness can strike at any time. If someone has hurt us and we haven't acknowledged it, hormonal imbalances can pull this unresolved issue to the forefront, making the flow of tears feel overwhelming and without end. If you have difficulty crying, your sadness may then express itself as rage. Learning how to "let it all hang out" when you need to cry can be very healing. If you repress your sadness, it will eventually overpower you and hit at a time when you least expect it. By identifying those issues that you're sad about, and then setting time aside to let your tears flow, you can begin to control your moods.

Not feeling our feelings is only one piece of the puzzle. Many of us also live lifestyles that create a breeding ground for PMS symptoms.

Lifestyle Remedies for Surviving PMS

— **Decrease caffeine, alcohol, salt, tobacco, and meat intake.** Caffeine can increase PMS symptoms. Caffeinated teas, coffee, sodas, and chocolates can contribute to blood-sugar imbalances, increasing the cravings for sugary junk foods. These foods create stress on the body and affect your emotional well-being. Breast tenderness is a common complaint from women who have PMS. This condition usually occurs a week before the onset of menstruation. Caffeine consumption can increase breast tenderness.

Alcohol interferes with blood-sugar levels because it's full of sugar. Many women suffer from hypoglycemic symptoms during PMS. Alcohol can intensify hypoglycemia, aggravating already existing PMS difficulties. Finally, both alcohol and caffeine are drastic diuretics. Such extreme action on the body exacerbates PMS symptoms.

Excessive salt intake can produce water retention. I always want salty popcorn two weeks before I start my period, but if I give in to this craving, I suffer dearly with bloating and swelling. Get in the habit of reading all of the labels on food products. If "salt" or "sodium" is found at the beginning of the "ingredients listed," avoid the product until after you've started menstruating.

Nicotine can constrict blood vessels and contribute to headaches. If you smoke, try to cut back on the nicotine content in the cigarettes you use two weeks before you begin your period.

In this country, it's common knowledge that the beef and poultry industry uses growth hormones when producing its products. The hormones in meats are generally unhealthy for us. For women, these additives are thought to contribute to PMS. If you're a meat eater, cut down on your meat intake, and try to purchase hormone-free products.

— **Moderate exercise.** A 30-minute brisk walk is a great example of moderate exercise. Several quick laps around the neighborhood can assist in relieving PMS symptoms. Comparisons have been made between women with PMS who exercise and those who do not. The results indicate that moderate (notice I said "moderate") exercise dramatically reduces PMS problems.

— **Try something new.** There are many alternative health practices that have proven to be useful for the woman suffering from PMS. My two favorites are massage and chiropractic adjustments. A good massage from a qualified caregiver can assist in reducing water retention, cramping, and mood swings. If my PMS is especially difficult, I have found that an adjustment from my chiropractor friend Judy does the trick. Some sufferers have found relief with acupuncture and acupressure. The needles used in acupuncture are extremely thin, and I have never felt pain during a treatment. Acupressure can also be very useful in relieving PMS.

You can learn how to apply acupressure to yourself by picking up one of the many books on this topic at your local bookstore. My favorite is *Acupressure Step by Step: The Oriental Way to Health,* by Jacqueline Young.

— **Meditation.** For many women, PMS can create mental confusion and emotional overload. Learning how to take the time to close your eyes and meditate for five minutes, three times a day, can help keep you centered. There are several different ways to meditate. Lying down and listening to a tape of ocean waves crashing on to a shoreline is most soothing. The rhythmic flow of the waves lowers both your heart rate and your blood pressure. Some women have found that visualizing color can be of great help. If you're feeling depressed, pick your favorite color and imagine yourself being encased in this hue. Color therapists believe that coral shades will improve the mood. For me, green lifts my depression. Experiment by visualizing different colors until you find one that feels right for you.

If we take the time to make the lifestyle changes necessary to remedy PMS, we will discover that these shifts in behavior will, in general, have a positive impact on the quality of our living experience. With this in mind, it's important to recognize that lifestyle also involves nutritional well-being. With PMS, our nutritional health is of paramount importance.

Nutritional and Herbal Support for Shifting Hormones

We live in a stressed-out society. Women of the new millennium continue to wear a number of hats: mother, worker, wife, lover, nurturer, taxi driver, comforter, healer, and more. As a result of this hectic way of life, we're not always diligent about our own nutritional well-being. As we've seen in the **Lifestyle** section, the foods we put in our body directly affect

PMS symptoms. Let's take a look at a few more nutritional tips for reducing PMS symptoms.

— **Watch what you eat.** Let's begin with keeping those blood-sugar levels regulated. Limit refined carbohydrates such as sugars and white-flour products. Because these items are easily absorbed into the system, they force blood-sugar levels to shoot up too quickly. After this, levels drop off quickly. This seesaw action can create intense mood swings. Instead, consume a diet rich in vegetables. Salads, cooked green leafy foods, carrot juices, and carrot sticks are full of necessary vitamins and minerals. Experiment with cooking different vegetable dishes. If you're a meat eater, put a small amount of hormone-free meat into a dish that primarily consists of stir- fried vegetables. Protein is very important, and it's not only found in meat. Did you know that vegetable protein from legumes and soy can be very beneficial? Tasty soy milk can be found in most grocery stores, and learning how to cook with tofu can be a great deal of fun. Tofu and soy products also contain soy isoflavones. These nutrients are especially beneficial for female health. Speaking of soy, soy nuts are very nutritious. I like to sprinkle them on top of my salads and baked potatoes.

Fish provides a good source of protein. In combination with vegetables, fish can assist in regulating hormone levels by encouraging the excretion of excess estrogen from the body.

Watch out for those saturated and partially hydrogenated fats found in meat products, mayonnaise, salad dressings, margarine, and packaged baked goods. Aside from being unhealthy, they're used by the body to produce prostaglandins. As mentioned earlier, if the body is high in prostaglandin hormones, this can contribute to PMS.

— **Let's supplement.** Not very many of us have time for the perfect diet. As a result, many women suffer from PMS symptoms because of nutritional deficiencies. In order for our hormones to successfully do what nature intended, we must be nutritionally fit. Essential vitamins and minerals are necessary to keep hormone levels on keel. If you're not taking a good, organically based multivitamin, begin doing so as soon as possible. Refer to Appendix II to determine what vitamins and minerals should be in a good multivitamin.

— PMS symptoms can result from **magnesium** deficiencies. Magnesium is a mineral that's necessary for the transmission of nerve impulses, and is essential for proper function of the nervous system. The mineral relaxes the nerves and relieves tension. As such, it's useful in promoting sleep. A lack of this mineral can produce heart palpitations, leg cramps, and fluid retention. To ensure proper health, 300–800 mg of magnesium per day is recommended. Check your multivitamin for magnesium content, and then supplement with magnesium aspartate or citrate. Take magnesium supplements with calcium at night to improve sleep.

— **How about some gamma-linoleic acid (GLA)?** GLA is necessary for women and has been found to reduce PMS symptoms such as breast tenderness, moodiness, and general soreness. Supplementing with oils containing GLA can solve these difficulties. **Evening primrose oil, borage oil, flaxseed oil, and black currant oil** are good sources for this nutrient. For PMS, begin by taking 500 mg of one of these oils per day. Do this for one month. Increase the dosage to 1,000 mg for the second month, and to 1,500 mg for the third month. If this doesn't work, you can take 1,000 mg two times per day the following month. Once you find a dose that works for you, maintain this dosage on a daily basis. Along with this supplement, you will need 400–600 IU of **Vitamin E** per day. Vitamin E oil will also help alleviate PMS symptoms such as headaches, insomnia, breast soreness, and moodiness. Check the Vitamin E content in your multivitamin and supplement if necessary.

(**Note:** If you're on a blood-thinning medication, check with your health-care provider before using this vitamin.)

— **Bring on the Vitamin C.** Want to get rid of the extra estrogen that's creating a hormonal imbalance in your system? Bring on the "C." Vitamin C is able to do this, thus reducing PMS. Extra C also helps the body during times of stress, and PMS is stressful. Research has shown that cells bathed in Vitamin C are more resistant to illness. Taking 1,000 mg of Vitamin C per day, divided into three doses, will keep a body healthy.

(**Note:** Some people suffer from an iron-overloading condition called "hemochromatosis." If you have this disease or if a member of your family suffers from hemochromatosis, talk to your health-care provider before increasing Vitamin C doses. Vitamin C assists the body in absorbing iron, and the last thing a person with hemochromatosis needs is more iron.)

— **Speaking of iron, can we talk?** If you're concerned about iron, have a cup of Cream of Wheat cereal topped with raisins for breakfast in the morning, or a nice spinach salad with sunflower seeds for lunch. These food products provide a good source of iron.

— **Give me a "B" . . . B complex, that is.** Even though your multivitamin contains B vitamins, supplementing with **Vitamin B complex** during those PMS days is not such a bad idea. Because B vitamins help take care of the nervous system, they also assist us in handling stress. B6 works with hormonal function and is very important. It's recommended that the multivitamin is taken in the morning, followed by the B complex at lunch.

— **A little acidophilus goes a long way.** Some nutritional experts have suggested that acidophilus bacteria is useful for

PMS because it normalizes the bowels. With normal bowels, not only is constipation no longer a problem, but estrogen is not as readily reabsorbed into the intestines. Reabsorbed estrogens can add to hormonal imbalance.

(**Note:** If you're allergic to lactose in dairy products, look for a "lactose-free" acidophilus, and take as directed on the label.)

A healthy diet can significantly reduce the physical and emotional stress of PMS. PMS takes a toll on the vitamins and minerals stored in your body. Recharging your physical temple with foods that are good for you will help you wade through those tough days.

Now that we've tackled nutrition, it's important to turn to herbs. Gifts from the world of medicinal plants have been used for centuries by women all around the world. The women of today can learn a lot from our sisters of days gone by.

— Bloating and water retention—not a girl's best friend. Water retention creates a number of PMS symptoms. To remedy this situation, let's first examine **couch grass.** Once used by Pliny (A.D. 23–79) for kidney stones and poor urine flow, couch grass has enjoyed a long history as a gentle diuretic. Aside from being a diuretic herb, it also possesses demulcent characteristics. This means that it's soothing on the system. Couch grass can be found in tea bags at the health food store. Use as directed on the label, or drink three cups of tea per day to reduce water retention.

Every once in a while, I find myself in a part of the world where I'm away from my herbs, unprepared for PMS water retention. During those times, I've found relief from the wonderful citrus fruit, **lemon.** For relief from water retention, I will drink 1–2 tablespoons of fresh lemon juice in a cup of warm water upon awakening in the morning.

— Back to blood-sugar levels. Because blood-sugar levels greatly contribute to our physical and emotional state of being, it's important to revisit this topic. My favorite green algae herb food, **spirulina,** works wonders on restoring healthy blood sugar. Be sure to purchase the tablets and use as directed. **Gentian,** a pretty plant native to the high Alps, has been growing in herbalists' gardens for centuries. Known for its ability to assist in controlling blood-sugar levels, Gentian is also useful in aiding the digestive system in absorbing many nutrients, including Vitamin B12 and iron. As a result, the herb is recommended to women with heavy bleeding during menstruation. Use in tincture or tea form as directed.

(**Note:** If you have an ulcer or acid indigestion, do not use this herb.)

— **Balancing those hormones.** Women have been using many different herbs for female hormonal problems for ages, and Vitex agnus-castus is one of these remedies. Once thought to reduce sexual desire, monks used to chew the berries of this plant in the hopes of decreasing their libido. No, you will not lose your sexual desire if you use Vitex, but you might be able to lessen PMS symptoms. Take as directed in tablet form first thing in the morning. Two months of consistent, continual use of this herb is necessary before results are noticed.

— **Oh, yes, cramp relief.** Cramping before the start of a period is a common complaint voiced by women experiencing PMS. **Crampbark** comes by its name for a reason. This Native American remedy was used by the Meskwaki people to relieve cramping in the body, and now we, too, can take advantage of this herb. Excessive contraction of the uterus can create excruciating pain, not only during PMS, but also once the period begins. Crampbark in capsule form can reduce cramping. Use as directed on the label. Crampbark also has sedative abilities, since it soothes the nervous system. **Red raspberry** tea will relax the uterus and alleviate cramping. Red raspberry leaf tea bags can be found at your local health food store.

— **Anxiety and those awful heart palpitations.** Nothing can be more disturbing at night when trying to get to sleep than the thumping of heart palpitations. **Motherwort** is a useful herb for females, and it has long been considered a heart remedy. For the woman suffering from PMS, this herb will not only lessen heart palpitations, but also produce a gentle state of relaxation, without drowsiness. Motherwort will also stimulate the muscles of the uterus and is useful for treating delayed periods.

(**Note:** Because of its uterine-stimulating properties, this herb should never be used during heavy periods or pregnancy.)

— **Stress and nervousness.** For PMS, nothing relieves stress better than **skullcap** tea, glycerin tincture, or capsules. This herb was routinely utilized by Native Americans for menstrual difficulties. Cherokee Indian women have used this herb for many years to relieve breast soreness and to stimulate delayed menstruation. Take as directed, three times a day. If you're taking a pharmaceutical antidepressant, tranquilizer, or muscle relaxant, do not use this herb.

PMS does not have to rule your life. If you address every area of your being, you can reclaim your physical, emotional, and spiritual self. By taking the time to care for your psychological, lifestyle, and nutritional needs, the difficulties of PMS can become a distant memory.

Norma felt just awful. She couldn't believe she had reacted so strongly to her family. *Bubbles . . . silly soap bubbles. My behavior was so out of line!* she thought as she washed her face with cold water. After she dried herself off, she made her way to her daughter's bedroom. Janie was lying on her bed, redoing her smudged nail polish. Sitting down on the bed, Norma put her arm around her oldest child and said, "I am so sorry for screeching at you like a madwoman." Janie then reached over to her dresser and handed her mother a pamphlet titled "Herbal Remedies for Women."

"What's this?" Norma asked.

"Mom, you have the most serious PMS ever! During this time, haven't you noticed we all kind of tiptoe around you?"

Looking at the pamphlet, Norma thought, *Out of the mouths of babes . . . guess it's time for me to do something about this!*

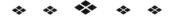

Chapter eighteen

MENOPAUSE: IT ISN'T A MENTAL ILLNESS

It was freezing outside. Absolutely bone-chilling. The sun had been down since 3:30 that afternoon, and by 6 o'clock, the stars glittered brightly against the dark sky like angel dust gently tossed to the four corners of the universe. In spite of the cold, Alaska really was magnificent at night. After trudging through knee-deep snow for what seemed like an eternity, my women friends and I were at our destination. The small house was buried in ice, but once inside, the heat of a roaring fire warmed us from head to toe. Women of all ages had gathered for this occasion. Gray-haired 85-year-olds were easily conversing with a pretty 20-year-old crowd. The room was buzzing with discussion ranging from the birthing of babies to the importance of maintaining femininity in the business world. Suddenly, our host clapped her hands and said, "Women, it's time."

Each woman was given a candle. With the lights dim, the slow burn of the fire, and the glowing wicks, the room took on an otherworldly appearance. One by one, each person, young and old, was asked to step forward and honor the women in her life who had made a difference. When my turn came, I shared thoughts about the invaluable love of a grandmother, the traumatic death of my mother, and the gentle touch of the many women who are in my life today.

After everyone had spoken, our host led a pretty middle-aged woman into the center of the room and said, "We're here to celebrate the many changes Katie has been experiencing over the last several years. These changes have made her wiser, more tolerant, and spiritual. Sadly, our culture not only belittles this major life experience, but then discards us because we're not brimming with youth. It's as if society believes that once the blood has stopped flowing, we're no longer of use. In ancient cultures, this change of life was celebrated. The menopausal woman was ceremoniously moved from the role of Mother to the time-honored rank of wise woman or Crone. The Crone was revered, respected, and sought out for her life experience and wisdom by men and women alike. In days gone by, she was a leading member of her community. It's time for us as women to rekindle this ancient observance. By celebrating every change of life, from the onset of menstruation to virginal deflowering, the experience of motherhood, and finally menopause, we can begin to empower ourselves as women. Katie is now postmenopausal, and she can rightfully claim the honored title of Crone."

Menopause is not a disease or a mental illness, but it can often be misdiagnosed as such. This is because the hormones estrogen and progesterone affect a number of bodily functions from brain chemistry to proper bone function. The heart, liver, and the body's internal thermostat also depend on estrogen. While a woman is bearing children, these hormones are essential for her health. Once she has moved past this stage of life, it doesn't make sense for the body to continue churning up energy for reproductive purposes. Contrary to popular belief, Mother

Nature was very wise in providing the female body with the ability to pause or end the menses (menopause). Since the body no longer requires the great stores of energy that were required for the reproductive years, why should the physical stress of the monthly menstrual cycle continue? Menopause actually saves on the "wear and tear" of the body.

Most women are unaware that this incredible transition begins 10 to 15 years before the actual advent of menopause. During this time, the ovaries gradually cease producing estrogen. Actual menopause begins when ovulation stops. With this, the production of estrogen and progesterone by the ovaries comes to an end. During this time, some women experience no symptoms, while others can have mood swings; flushes; fatigue; heart palpitations; dryness of the skin, hair, and vaginal area; depression; or insomnia. With proper diet, nutrition, and emotional support, most of these unpleasant side effects can be minimized and even eliminated. If a woman ignores this life change and does not take care of herself, she can be at risk for osteoporosis and cardiovascular disease. Physically, menopause does not have to be a frightening, dreaded experience. It's a chance for women to really gain an appreciation and acceptance of the miracle and wisdom of the female body.

Even though estrogen levels drop off rather sharply after menopause, this hormone does not entirely disappear. Other organs in the body take over from the ovaries and begin producing small amounts of estrogen. For this reason, it's extremely important to nutritionally support these organs. Research has even suggested that progesterone may be more important than estrogen. Utilizing foods and herbs that contain natural progesterone can provide effective relief from many menopausal symptoms and even stimulate the body's production of estrogen. The menopause transition can last for up to five years. Once a woman hasn't had a menstrual cycle for a year, she's considered postmenopausal. Free from monthly periods, PMS, and the fear of unwanted pregnancy, emotionally she's more able to direct her attention toward self-growth and exploration. In order to have a successful menopause, the psychology of this experience must be examined.

The Psychology of Menopause

— **A healing time.** Menopause can be an emotionally productive time. This phase of life has the potential for being one of the most challenging, exciting, and rewarding times of a woman's life. If handled properly, this process may produce profound gifts in the long run. Initially, the emotional adjustment of recognizing that the childbearing years are over can initiate grieving. If this grief is ignored, it will be difficult to embrace and enjoy the adventure of the next phase of life. For those women who fear aging, menopause can be an emotional struggle. Feeling worthless, unattractive, or that life has come to an end because children have grown up and moved on are emotions related to unaddressed grief. Menopause can also trigger unresolved life problems such as a divorce, death, loss of a job, or even childhood issues. The great distraction to healing from these issues involves focusing on not having a youthful appearance or feeling less desirable by society. Experiencing appropriate grief and dealing directly with the associated emotions allows a woman to eventually appreciate herself as a mature, wise, postmenopausal female.

— **Grieving is an art.** Knowing how to grieve is essential to developing a sense of spirituality. Using the emotions that menopause produces can be a stepping-stone to healthy grieving and healing. To grieve the loss of reproduction, it's useful to gather up pictures of the self from puberty to the motherhood years. Include pictures of children when they were young and in their baby years. Do you remember the fear of birthing the first baby or the insecure moments of being a young woman with very little life experience? Put these photographs in chronological order and review them. Let the emotions rise to the surface and express them. Cry at the loss of youth and the baby years of childhood, or get angry about developing wrinkles and pound on a stack of pillows. Write letters to the body, God, or Mother Nature about the grief, sadness, or rage of losing the use of the reproductive organs. If necessary, allow the confusion of having identified the self only as mother or nurturer to rise to consciousness. Experience the fear of not knowing where to go from here. These intense emotions will not last for long if they're expressed. If anger, sadness, and fear are ignored, they will manifest as clinical depression.

— **Unresolved life issues** triggered by the emotions of menopause are a signal to use this time to *clean up the past.* Ignoring these issues will make menopause an extremely negative experience. A good therapist can nurture a woman through these issues. During this time, such an experience can provide a great deal of physical and emotional relief. Talking about menopause with other women is also very important.

Women of the past went through menopause alone and in shame. Some women have even been hospitalized for certain emotional or physical conditions that were related to menopause. Not understanding that these conditions were normal and necessary for the body's long-term survival left women feeling as though something was wrong with them. It's very important to talk to other menopausal women and also to mothers, grandmothers, and aunts who have already been through menopause. Most women go through menopause at the age that their mothers did. Symptoms of menopause from mother to daughter are usually very similar. Knowing this can provide a great deal of relief for the woman approaching the menopause years. Joking about hot flashes with a friend can be normalizing, and it will reduce the fear that this transition can produce. Reading positive books and literature on the menopausal process can also be of benefit.

Menopause does not have to be a lonely experience. Reaching out to others can make all the difference in the world. The more information a woman has about her body and its functions, the better prepared she will be for its many changes.

Essential Lifestyle Remedies for Surviving and Learning from Menopause

Lifestyle changes are so important for the woman who is menopausing. This particular life experience can serve as a wake-up call for the professional nurturer who has spent her life taking care of others at the expense of herself. Below are some of the lifestyle changes that must be addressed.

— **Exercise.** Regular exercise, not obsessive exercise, helps the body remain fit and supple. Appropriate exercise can assist in maintaining bone density, reducing the risk for osteoporosis. Because the risk of bone loss is greatest in the first few years after menopause, developing a healthy habit of brisk walking and light weight lifting can work wonders for the body. Emotionally, exercise counters depression and "blue moods" by stimulating the brain, releasing mood-enhancing endorphin. Modern dance, yoga, and stretching exercises can reacquaint a woman with her body and teach her how to appreciate it.

(**Note:** Women who over-exercise and are underweight are more at risk for osteoporosis. Estrogen and other related hormones are stored in body fat. Because underweight women tend to have less body fat, they will have less estrogen in their system after menopause.)

— **Sex, sex, sex.** A woman recently called my office and asked, "Will I hate sex once I start to menopause?"

To this, I chuckled and replied, "I don't think so. As a matter of fact, I've talked to a number of postmenopausal women who say that sex is better than ever." Just ask the 50-, 60-, 70-, and 80-year-olds who have visited my office. If anything, after this particular physical change, sex with a partner can finally be more spontaneous. Pregnancy is no longer a worry, and frequent sexual intercourse can relieve the vaginal dryness that can accompany menopause. As estrogen decreases, the lining of the vagina begins to thin, making the genital area more sensitive. By applying Vitamin E oil to the vaginal area, this intimate part of the body remains moist. Using KY Jelly or Vitamin E during intercourse can provide pleasure for the woman who may suddenly be experiencing dryness.

— **Loose, comfortable, layered clothing** made of cotton can make life more comfortable for the woman who is experiencing hot flushes or flashes. Hot flashes can be confusing if women are not educated about their purpose. Such flushes of body heat usually start at the head and work their way down, causing increased perspiration, often followed by chills. Many times women who breast-feed will experience hot flashes, and if this is the case, hot flashes during menopause will not be new or frightening. The hot flash is caused by the body's attempt to readjust to the hormonal changes that are taking place. It's important to note that estrogen is a natural temperature regulator for the body. It makes perfect sense that a drop in estrogen production would cause thermal swings. Menopause can be a time for a woman to create a "new look" for herself, one that isn't dictated by the fashion police and the modeling profession.

(**Note:** Smoking and alcohol consumption can trigger hot flashes.)

— **Discover the world of massage.** A good massage can leave the mind at peace and the body totally relaxed. Mixing sweet almond oil with medicinal herbs specifically used to alleviate menopausal symptoms will leave the skin moist and the hormones balanced. The essential oil **geranium** is a wonderful hormonal balancer, while the oil of the **rose** is useful for tonifying and detoxing the reproductive organs. When feeling emotionally out of sorts, **chamomile** or **neroli** oil can be massaged into the body to relieve anxiety or depression.

— **Drink plenty of liquids.** Now is the time to reduce caffeine intake and begin experimenting with herbal teas. Herbal teas can be calming, nutritious, and relaxing. Different fragrant, fruity-flavored herbs can be mixed to create new sensations for the taste buds, and their often appealing colors make them an asset to any meal. It's important to drink a minimum of two quarts of liquid a day to keep the skin and the mucous membranes moist. Caffeine dehydrates the body, intensifies mood swings, and can trigger hot flashes. Begin cutting back on the intake of caffeine in coffee by using a combination of decaffeinated and caffeinated beans. Cut down on caffeinated teas and sodas, and be sure to check foods for possible caffeine content. I recently discovered that my favorite chocolate yogurt was loaded with caffeine.

— **Alternative medicine** has a couple of remedies for the menopausal woman. **Homeopathy** has been used over the decades by women for menopausal symptoms. When applying this technique to improve the menopause experience, it's wise to follow the guidance of a qualified health-care provider. **Acupuncture** is an ancient technique that can be utilized in balancing out "chi," or life force energy. By rebalancing the hormonal system, a knowledgeable acupuncturist can alleviate heavy periods, poor memory and concentration, back pain, and improve skin tone. Acupuncture needles are very small, and they cause little or no discomfort.

By addressing the psychology of menopause, a woman can find this experience to be a time of growth and spiritual evolution. Emotionally and spiritually, women can begin to blossom into the people they were always meant to be. By changing her lifestyle, a woman can enhance her creativity, making this passage into the role of the "wise woman" an exciting one. Now it's time to investigate how nutrition and herbs can assist the menopausal woman in becoming a stronger, healthier individual.

Nutritional and Herbal Support for the Changing Female Body

— "If it grows, eat it. If it doesn't grow, don't eat it," says author Louise Hay. By putting whole, naturally nutritious foods into the body, a woman can eliminate a number of menopausal symptoms. Nutritionally supporting the body and those organs assisting in the hormonal changes taking place is essential. Follow the **Healthy Body/Well Mind Diet Plan** found in Appendix I, along with the **Supplement for Health** plan found in Appendix II. Then begin implementing the following nutritional and dietary suggestions.

- The adrenal glands produce small amounts of estrogen after menopause. As a result, it's important to nutritionally support these glands. Since the pituitary gland is the "chief in charge," or master gland controlling all other glands, it, too, must receive special attention. By removing caffeine from the diet, stress on these particular glands is decreased. Extra **Vitamin B5** is also needed for healthy adrenal function. Taking 100 mg of this powerful anti-stress vitamin, three times a day, can keep the adrenals working up to potential.

Vitamin B6, 50 mg three times a day, also relieves stress and minimizes water retention.

- Along with extremely spicy food, red meat should be cut out of the diet. Red meat, excessive sugar, and spicy foods make the blood more acidic, and this pulls calcium from the bones into the bloodstream. Also, too much meat in the diet can also trigger hot flashes. Utilizing more plant, bean, grain, and legume protein will lessen this burden on the body. Sugar is another hot-flash culprit, and it can create blood-sugar disruptions and mood swings that contribute to depression. By consuming a diet consisting mainly of fresh whole grains, raw vegetables, and fruits, along with a daily **spirulina tablet,** the blood-sugar levels will naturally stabilize.

- Research has shown that American women, in general, suffer from many more menopausal symptoms than do Japanese women. Interestingly, the reason for this is purely nutritional. Japanese women consume a great deal more **phytoestrogens** (plant estrogens) than do American women. Plant estrogens can be found in many yummy foods, including soybeans, tofu, and tofu products (ice cream-like desserts and tofu-based drinks) miso, flaxseeds, pomegranates, and dates. These substances act like the estrogen produced in the body. Hormone-like substances can also be found in whole grains, seeds, carrots, ripe bananas, apples, royal jelly, and bee pollen.

- **Vitamin E** has been touted as the elixir of youth by the media for years. Maybe there's some truth to this. This vitamin is essential for reducing hot flashes and other menopausal symptoms. It also keeps the reproductive organs healthy and the skin supple. Begin taking 500

IUs daily for several weeks. Then increase this up to 1,600 IUs per day, or until hot flashes have subsided. **Lecithin capsules** need to be taken with this vitamin because they're an emulsifier for Vitamin E. Lecithin will help Vitamin E do its job; 1,200 mg–1,300 mg of lecithin, taken three times a day before meals can aid Vitamin E in reducing hot flashes.

Evening primrose or **black currant seed oil pearls** are important supplements to consider because they, too, can assist in the production of estrogen in the body. As a result, they also help to relieve hot flashes. These two nutrients deserve several more "gold stars" because they have sedative and diuretic qualities. Evening primrose or black currant seed oil pearls should be taken as directed on the label. **Vitamin C** not only assists in fighting viruses and colds, but it, too, can fight off hot flashes. Vitamin C should also be increased during menopause. Take 5,000–10,000 mg of Vitamin C in three divided daily doses to reduce the burn of hot flashes.

- Bone loss is a great concern during and immediately after menopause. Taking care of the **calcium** needs of a woman in middle age will leave her with relatively strong bones for the golden years. Dairy foods; salmon sardines (with the bones); seafood; green, leafy vegetables; almonds; oats; blackstrap molasses; and tofu are just a few examples of the food sources rich in this mineral. **Calcium,** along with **magnesium,** relieves nervousness and irritability, and if taken at night, can aid in a good night's sleep. Taken as a daily supplement, use 2,200 mg of calcium with 500–1,000 mg of magnesium in a chelated form. The nutrient **boron** also enhances calcium absorption.

(**Note:** A total daily dose of boron should never exceed 3 mg.)

In addition, 50 mg of zinc taken on a daily basis not only protects against bone loss, but also reduces menopausal symptoms. (**Note:** Do not exceed a daily dose of 100 mg of zinc from all supplements. Finally, cut down on salt intake. Use onion and garlic to add flavor to food. Excessive use of salt can increase urinary excretion of calcium.)

- **Gamma-oryzanol** is a nutrient that is derived from rice bran. This particular nutrient has been shown to be particularly effective in controlling the uncomfortable side effects of menopause. Take as directed on the label.

Hormone Replacement Therapy

There's a great deal of controversy surrounding **hormonal replacement therapy (HRT)**. Because of the dangerous side effects associated with hormonal replacement treatments, any woman considering HRT should investigate all of the facts regarding the different types of hormones used in these programs. If a woman decides to use HRT, it's strongly suggested that she consider only truly natural estrogens such as Estropipate or Estradiol. Consult with a health-care provider who is dedicated to a more holistic approach of treatment and who is well informed on HRT.

Good nutrition is a major key to a healthy body during menopause. The more nutritionally fit a woman is at this time, the more likely she will be able to handle the many challenges that menopause can create. Accommodating the massive hormonal modifications that menopause can bring about depends on the body's ability to flow with these changes. The menopausal woman can be assured of a fairly smooth ride if she puts into her body only those food sources that work with this transitional process.

Let's now take a look at a few of the herbs recommended for women who have reached this life-changing milestone.

— The herb world is full of natural estrogen promoters. **Black cohosh,** also known as "squaw root," is an old Native American remedy for female problems. Research in Germany showed that the root of the black cohosh plant, in combination with the herb **St. John's wort,** was effective 78 percent of the time in treating many menopausal problems, especially hot flashes. St. John's wort is also useful for mild depression, but do not use it if you're currently taking traditional tranquilizers, antidepressants, or sleep medication.

Wild yam, a traditional remedy for female concerns in Central America, has wonderful hormonal properties. As a matter of fact, one of the ingredients in the root of the wild yam paved the way for the development of the first contraceptive pill. This herb is used by many women for its hormonal balancing abilities in herbal creams, tinctures, and decoctions.

Helonias, or **false unicorn,** is another herb specifically utilized by herbalists for female reproductive difficulties. False unicorn can be very beneficial during menopause, and this particular herb combines well with black cohosh.

The herb **agnus-castus** is a wonderful hormonal balancer. Researchers have been investigating this plant for more than 30 years, and they're well aware of the distinct hormonal effect that the golden-red berries have on the hormonal system. Other herbs to consider using as estrogen promoters are **raspberry** and **sarsaparilla.** Used as a tincture, the above herbs have been shown to be supportive of the hormones during menopause.

Many women complain of hot flashes during menopause. Sweet-smelling **sage,** once thought to ward off the evil eye, is also a hormonal stimulant. Its hormonal action is not completely understood, but this fragrant plant will reduce hot flashes and can help the body adapt to the hormonal changes menopause brings. For the relief of hot flashes, take this herb in an infusion three times a day or whenever a hot flash strikes.

(**Note:** Do not use sage medicinally if epileptic or pregnant.)

White willow, sacred to all deities of the Underworld in classic mythology, contains salicin, a constituent of aspirin. This herb also reduces sweating and can be used for hot flashes.

(**Note:** Do not use this herb if there's an allergic relation to aspirin.)

White peony, used medicinally for close to 1,500 years in China, has long been considered a woman's remedy and is also useful for hot flashes. If the menopausing woman is interested in experimenting with her creativity, she can make a **Hot Flash Brew** by taking equal parts of **sage, hawthorn tops,** and **black currant leaves,** and steeping them as a tea. It's suggested that two teaspoons of dried herbs be used for every cup of boiling water. This herbal combination must be used regularly over several months to completely alleviate hot flashes.

— Because **energy levels** are certain to drop periodically, maintaining vitality during this time is very important. Looking to the plant world, solutions can be found. Used regularly, **kombucha tea** has been found by many menopausal women to increase energy levels and reduce menopausal symptoms. **Kelp tablets** can also be used to increase energy levels. Taken daily, they can give the body an energizing boost.

— **Emotionally,** menopause can be a stressful time. For some women, mood swings, anxiety, and depression can become a problem. Instead of turning to often-toxic psychotropic medications, try a few herbs from Mother Nature's garden. **Skullcap,** worn as a charm by wives to protect their husbands from other women during medieval times, is a wonderful herb for reducing anxiety. Used by herbalists as a remedy for calming the nervous system, this herb can be taken as a tincture, infusion, or in capsule form. (**Note:** Do not use this herb with prescription medication, especially traditional tranquilizers and antidepressants.) **Oats** are also mildly antidepressive. This well-known nutritious grain can increase energy levels and has been used for centuries to treat depression and nervous exhaustion. By regularly including oats in the diet, a menopausal woman can improve her mood and vitality. Insomnia, another symptom of menopause, can plague a woman, leaving her exhausted and blurry-eyed the next morning. The sweet aromatic **German chamomile** herb has long been valued for its use in relieving nervousness and irritability. Not only does it promote sleep in adults, but it can be used safely with children as well. (**Note:** Do not use if there's an allergy to common ragweed.) **Kava kava** is also useful for sleeplessness.

— In order to **protect the bones** from osteoporosis, herbs can be included in the diet to increase **calcium** intake. Drink three cups of **chickweed, nettle,** and **dandelion** tea per day. At one time, nettle was carried to frighten off ghosts and wrongdoing spirits, but today, the main evil it wards off is bone deterioration.

Menopause is not a disease, but a natural, normal transition every woman will eventually go through. Over the last century, our culture has become more obsessed with youth. As a result, menopause is looked upon with dread by most women. Traditional medicine has fueled this belief by insinuating that without the use of synthetic hormones, life for the menopausal woman is essentially over. As one woman told me, "Menopause, from what my doctor says, is a real bummer." This perception is totally false. Menopause is actually an exciting passageway into the second half of a woman's life.

When the Croning ceremony was over, the group stood in a circle, held hands, and gave thanks in song and prayer to God for the wisdom of Mother Nature. Afterward, I found myself sitting next to a couple of 70-year-old women. One had the loveliest, blue-gray hair. Looking at her I thought to myself, *If she can have long locks at her age, well then, so can I.*

After this revelation, I turned to her and asked, "Seriously, is menopause scary?"

She laughed and then replied, "What on earth is there to be afraid of? If you don't fight it, and work *with* the body instead of against it, the 'change,' as my mother used to call it, can be one of life's greatest adventures." She slowly looked around the room at the other wise women who had been listening to our conversation. One by one, they returned her gaze with a knowing wink, nod, or smile.

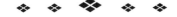

Chapter nineteen

AGING: A NATURAL CONSEQUENCE OF LIVING

Her lovely dark hair was sprinkled with just a bit of gray, and wild curls framed her olive-toned face. "I hate getting old. Hate it!" she raged as she pounded away on a stack of pillows. "Everything goes to hell in a handbasket!" Whack, went the red plastic bat. "When I go jogging in the morning, these thin, young, pretty creatures go galloping past me; and I feel old, decrepit, and unattractive." Whack. Whack. My 50-year-old client, Eleanor, was really giving the pillows in my office a workout. "I hate looking at myself in the mirror." Whack, went the bat one more time. "Do you know that I wasn't given a promotion because of my age?" Whack. Whack. Whack.

At this point, Eleanor was really getting into her anger. "I know it's against the law to discriminate against age, but that's what happened to me." Whack. Whack. Whack. "Instead of promoting me, the higher-ups gave the position to some young, good-looking kid who's still wet behind the ears!" she screamed.

After much yelling and pounding, Eleanor started to cry. "During my lifetime, I've raised a family, worked my fingers to the bone, and how does society reward me? As soon as the first wrinkle appears, I'm treated as though I'm useless and as if I don't have a brain in my head. When I was young, I respected my elders. I didn't treat them like this!" Eleanor then pushed several strands of hair out of her face, grabbed a tissue, and blew her red nose.

"You know," she continued, "my mother hated aging. She would never have admitted it, but I always knew she absolutely hated it. Mother avoided funerals, death, dying, and would never talk about such things with me." Eleanor reached for her cup of herbal tea and took a sip. "The bottom line is that my poor mother hated aging because she was afraid of dying. Hell, when she was on her deathbed, she still wouldn't discuss it. I don't want to spend the rest of my years fearing lost youth and death such as she did. Yes, society is discriminating against me, and believe me, I'm going to do something about that. But I'm also starting to think that part of my problem just might be tied to my difficulty in looking at death. What do you think, Doc?"

Eleanor was right on target about a number of things. First of all, today's society does not appear to openly respect and appreciate the wisdom of the elderly, but, thankfully, this group is fighting back—politically, socially, and even economically. Second, youth and beauty *are* highly valued. I always laugh when a television advertisement has a gorgeous 20-something-year-old woman selling aging cream. The media uses youth to sell everything from cars to colas. In our culture, we're all constantly bombarded with images of youth. Also, we live in a "death phobic" society. The ill are typically relegated to hospitals and nursing homes, while the dying often pass on alone.

Generations of the past appreciated the wisdom of the more mature, saw death as a natural part of the living experience, and grew old gracefully. Today's tendency to buy into the media's obsession with youth, while at the same time dreading the aging process, is a sad commentary on our society. We need to recognize that the second half of our lives can be a great adventure. Life doesn't have to end with a few gray hairs. Here are a few psychological issues to consider with regard to healthy aging.

The Psychology of Aging

— **Give yourself permission to grieve.** As we pass through one phase of life to the next, it's important to say good-bye before we move on. Too many people make the mistake of dismissing the grief that accompanies us as we age. If we ignore this, we will lose out on the many gifts aging has to offer. Here is a visualization I use with each birthday.

Close your eyes and visualize yourself in your childhood years, during your teenage days, as a young adult in your 20s and 30s, middle age, and, if appropriate, in your later years. While visualizing each stage of your life, ask yourself, "What did I really like about myself physically, emotionally, and spiritually at each of the stages in my life?" While doing so, notice how you feel. Go ahead and cry if you need to. It's okay to admit that you miss how your body looked at 20, or to grieve about days gone by. This is healthy. This is how we let go of our youth. By doing so, you will be able to embrace the years ahead.

Next, ask yourself, "Did I grow and mature from the many lessons I encountered this year?" Meditate on the challenges you've faced thus far, and ask, "How have these experiences made me a more complete person?"

Finally, imagine bringing all of these different images of yourself into one room for a party. It's time to celebrate the many different aspects of your life. You are the host of this celebration, so create a party environment that pleases you. Now visualize yourself greeting your guests. Imagine going to each of these separate parts of you and embracing them. Thank them for being a part of your life, and tell them that they will always be with you. After this exercise, open your eyes and write about your feelings. Share this with a therapist, spiritual advisor, or close friend.

A number of elders over 100 years old were once asked, "What's your secret to living so long?" Their collective response was, "You roll with the punches." These centenarians knew how to grieve life's losses and move on. Just last year, my 105-year-old neighbor, John W. Harris, passed away. I must tell you, I learned a great deal about "rolling with the punches" from this wise old man. I'm glad he was my friend.

— **Looking death in the eye.** There's an old proverb that goes something like this: "If you avoid death, you can't totally embrace life." As mentioned earlier, our own attitudes about death can often dictate our approach toward aging. Core beliefs about death and dying are usually based on childhood experiences. Close your eyes, and visualize your parents and grandparents. Ask yourself, "How did they feel about death? Could they talk about it? In my family, what is it like when someone dies? As a child, did I go to funerals? How was death and dying explained to me?" So many people in our culture today fear death. If our parents were uncomfortable with aging, dying, or death, we will have difficulty with it, too.

Many aging issues are tied up with unresolved concerns about death. In order to free ourselves from these constraints, we must be willing to look death in the eye. Here is a great visualization for confronting this issue.

Close your eyes and take several deep breaths. Visualize yourself lying in a bed, dying. Your family is with you, and your favorite pet is at by your side. You're telling your family good-bye, so cry if you need to. Next, imagine that you see a loving deceased relative, angel, or any other concept of a Higher Power (God, Jesus, Buddha, Moses, and so on) standing at the foot of your bed. This being is here to take you to the Other Side or Afterlife. Visualize taking the hand of this guide, following him or her to a tunnel, bridge, sea, or river. As you make your way through the tunnel, across the river, or over the bridge, you will see a number of loved ones who have already made this trip, waiting for you on the other side. Imagine these deceased loved ones embracing and welcoming you. Open your eyes, and write out your experience.

Looking at the psychology of aging can provide us with a great deal of relief. As we age, our psychological well-being can also be greatly enhanced by a number of lifestyle changes.

Lifestyle Remedies to Keep Us Healthy As We Age

— **Premature aging: It's not a necessity!** The baby-boomer generation is slowly aging. In just a few years, one out of every six adults in this country will be a senior citizen. Yes, a whole bunch of us are trekking down the path toward our golden years. How can we age gracefully? By being aware of what aging is. First of all, aging isn't a sickness. Although society treats it as such, in actuality, this is a normal, physiological process. What makes us sick often has to do with the lifestyle we're living. Living an unhealthy lifestyle will produce premature aging.

Many people age prematurely for several reasons. Weight, smoking, and other toxins appear to be the biggest culprits. Interestingly, those segments of the population involved with religions that discourage the use of excessive alcohol, caffeine, tobacco, and recreational drugs appear to have long life spans. Members of the Mormon Church abstain from all of the above and have the longest, healthiest life spans of any religious group in the United States.

When I see people my age (40s) smoking, they usually look much older than I do. Smoking really does a number on the skin. Excessive sun exposure can also wreak havoc on the complexion by promoting free radicals. Free radicals damage cell structure, and this is thought to promote premature aging. Cell production slows down as we move on in years, and as a result, we need to protect our healthy cells.

Food additives, certain drugs, alcohol, and tobacco can also contribute to cellular damage. Excessive weight creates more work for our organs, causing breakdown in these systems. It's important to do what we can to maximize our potential for a healthy life by minimizing damage to our internal organs and cells. If you're living an unhealthy lifestyle, now is the time to do something about it.

— **The essentials.** We can do several things to improve how we age. Proper rest, relaxation, and enjoyable hobbies can reduce stress. Excessive stress lowers the immune system, making us vulnerable to disease and illness. Nobody is going to put time aside for you to relax. You must make the time to "chill out" yourself. If you keep running and don't slow down, life will pass you by. And remember this saying: *Premature aging and an early death is nature's way of telling you to slow down.*

Get regular exercise and move those limbs. Swimming, folk dancing, tai chi, walking, weight lifting—do anything to keep the body limber. Active, enjoyable physical exercise reduces stress. Physical activity also moves much-needed oxygen to the tissues in the body, and this slows down aging. My friend Mr. Harris was still walking around the block when he was 100 years old.

The moral of this message is: Excessive stress can put you into an early grave. Take time to unwind, and mellow out every day. Also, be sure to give your body the nightly "recharge" it needs with seven to eight hours of sleep.

— **Read, read, read.** Get a reality check on how those before you have aged. Reading the biography of someone you admire who lived a long healthy life—such as a celebrity, world or spiritual leader, or past historical figure—lets you know that your life is definitely not over. If an individual you respect has been able to live life to the fullest, so can you. Find a mentor, someone to model yourself after.

In both my family and my husband's, longevity is very common. Those family members who seem to be enjoying their 70s, 80s, and 90s continue to be socially involved with friends, family, the arts, education, religious groups, and civic activities. I know a couple of 80-year-olds who are in college. My mother-in-law studied Italian in her late 70s. Yes, if you exercise the brain, it will serve you well in later years.

— **Explore your spirituality.** In many cultures, life after 40 is seen as the most exciting time for spiritual exploration. Children have grown, financially, things have settled down, and work life is routine. Now is the moment to really investigate spiritual matters.

I have written a number of books, but I didn't start producing books of a spiritual nature until after I hit my 40s. In my recent book, *One Last Hug*, I explore a spiritual phenomenon that is close to my heart, deathbed visions (DBVs). When a person is dying, it's not uncommon for them to report visitations from deceased loved ones, angels, or religious figures. The goal of these deathbed visitations is to help the dying individual pass over.

Family members and loved ones at the deathbed also report experiencing deathbed visions. As my mother passed away in the hospital, across town I felt her leaving before I received verification that she had died. At the exact moment of her death, two other friends of mine also felt her pass. Like me, neither of them were at the hospital with her. For me, this experience removed any fear of death.

Another friend of mine, Judy Guggenheim, has written a book about after-death communications, or ADCs, called *Hello from Heaven*. ADCs can come in the form of seeing, hearing, or feeling a deceased loved one's presence. The day after my father-in-law passed, my husband saw him sitting in our den. Although Pop had been ill for some time, he now looked whole, healthy, and happy. This after-death communication convinced my husband that life does not end with the death of the physical body.

Explore the many different written works available on spiritual development, religious philosophies, and life-after-death research at your local library or bookstore. By the way, books found at used bookstores can save you a bundle of money.

No matter how old you are, there's still a lot out there to learn. Take the time to explore the "unknown." What you discover will not only surprise you, but might erase any fear you have about aging, death, and dying.

Approaching aging from a holistic point of view forces us to examine every area of our life. Not only do we need to change our thinking and lifestyle, but we must also look more closely at how our physical state of being can be improved. It's well known that many nutritional deficiencies contribute to premature aging. Let's see what we can do to keep this from happening.

Nutritional and Herbal Support for a Physically Fit Body and Healthy Mind

— **You must change your eating habits.** As my husband approached 50, he noticed something. If he ate high-fat, greasy foods for dinner, he paid for it dearly. After a weekend of burgers, fries, fried fish, poorboy sandwiches, and twice-baked potatoes, he thought he was suffering from heart failure on Monday morning. Once our doctor friend, Bob, checked him out with a variety of tests, he announced, "Michael, you can't eat like a 20-year-old anymore."

Would you believe that a third to one-half of all health problems for those 65 years or older are related to nutrition and diet? What we do and don't put into our bodies becomes extremely important.

As we age, we need fewer calories. Research has suggested that if we decrease our calories as we age, our life span will be increased. Does this mean that you should go on some celebrity-endorsed diet? No. Although we must cut calories, we want each calorie to be nutritionally full.

The high-fat foods of youth that once may have given us a boost of energy now leave us lethargic, overweight, and even depressed. We must cut down on fats and decrease our intake of animal products. Research has shown that vegetarians live longer than meat eaters. Trappist monks practice a vegetarian diet, and they, as a group, have a long life span.

If you're a meat eater, follow a few simple rules: Instead of fried fish or chicken, experiment with smaller baked portions. Grill small low-fat pieces of beef, or stir fry with a variety of colorful vegetables. Because protein products tend to take longer to digest, meats should be eaten earlier in the day.

With age, it's very important to increase the amount of raw and cooked vegetables we consume. Whole grains, oats, bran breads, and legumes can replace that hefty hunk of fat-riddled steak. This extra fiber helps keep the colon cleaned out. If we do not take care of the colon, we're at risk for suffering from illness and degenerative diseases.

Also, watch the sugar at night. As the years roll on, we often find that sugar products just before bed keep us awake. For nighttime snacks, grab a handful of low-fat crackers, a bagel, or some other type of complex carbohydrate. Complex carbohydrates will induce a relaxed state and make it easier for you to fall asleep at night.

Now is the time to increase your intake of garlic and onions. Not only does garlic assist your body in lowering cholesterol, but its antioxidant content fights those nasty free radicals. Garlic's sister, the onion, will also help lessen free radicals. Because garlic can cause heartburn, and onions can create gas, use these foods early in the day.

Finally, remember to take in six to eight glasses of liquid per day. Thirst often decreases as we age, but our requirements for good old H_2O must still be attended to. Herbal teas and fresh vegetable juices can provide a number of vitamins and minerals. To this day, I can still remember my grandmother's green pea juice. Yuck. May I suggest carrots, an apple, or a few strawberries instead? Try some green tea or grape juice for a boost of antioxidants. I have green tea for lunch and pure grape juice Popsicles at night. Remember, free radicals cause premature aging. Antioxidants will fight free radicals.

— **Malnutrition and aging.** For some of us, eating becomes more difficult as we age. As children move out of the house, many of us stop cooking nutritious meals for ourselves. When I'm at the store, it's not uncommon for me to be behind a 50-, 60-, or 70-year-old person at the checkout stand who has a basket full of doughnuts, chips, hot dogs, and sodas. These foods create degeneration and can lead to malnutrition. To remedy this problem, get out your Crockpot. Throw a bunch of veggies into it. Grab some of your favorite herbs; and top off with a vegetable, beef, or chicken broth. If you're a meat eater, add some diced skinned chicken, turkey, or fat-trimmed beef. Shrimp or fish will also add a wonderful flavor to this concoction. Let your creation cook on low for about eight hours, and then serve in a bowl with noodles or brown rice.

The juices from your simmered foods are full of vitamins, so spoon that into your bowl as well. Served with a simple salad and a hearty piece of whole-grain bread, this very nutritious meal is also easy to chew and digest. During the second half of life, there's no excuse for malnutrition. This will only happen if we neglect our nutritional needs.

— **Easily absorbed supplements.** As we age, the hydrochloric acid in our stomachs diminishes, making digestion more difficult. When this happens, we often find that we're not absorbing all of the nutrients from our foods. If we don't absorb the vitamins and minerals necessary for maintaining health, we're at risk for premature aging, physical degeneration, and illness. Eating five to six small meals, as opposed to three large meals per day, can lessen the burden on the digestive system. In addition, we may need to supplement our diet with certain vitamins and minerals. Here are just a few recommendations:

- **A multivitamin.** Because the stomach may have difficulty breaking down certain food products, care must be taken when choosing a vitamin supplement. If you're lacking in the hydrochloric acid needed to absorb foods, you may have trouble digesting many nutrient supplements. As with all of your supplements, make sure that your multivitamin is easily absorbed. It should also contain all 22 essential vitamins and 20 necessary minerals for good health. (See Appendix II.)

- Taking 90–100 mg of **Coenzyme Q10** is a great nutrient for maintaining the health of the heart, immune system, and circulatory system.

- Don't just drink grape juice, but enjoy the benefits of **grape seed extract.** This nutrient is a wonderful free-radical scavenger. Use as directed on the label.

- Both **Vitamins E and C** are powerful antioxidants. Although they will be in your multivitamin, you might want to add an extra dose of these nutrients; 5,000–6,000 mg daily of easily absorbed, buffered Vitamin C will protect the immune system and fight fatigue. Taking 800–1,000 mg of daily Vitamin E gives our cells added life by protecting cell membranes. Begin with a small dose of 300 mg, and then build up to 800–1,000 mg over a period of weeks.

  (**Note:** If you're on an anticoagulant medication or are going to be having surgery in the next few weeks, talk to your health-care provider before taking this supplement.)

- Blood-sugar levels often become an issue as we age. This can be rectified with **spirulina** or **chromium picolinate.** Take as directed on the label.

- If you want to give your brain a little boost and emulsify fat at the same time, get some **lecithin capsules.** Use as directed.

- We can take care of the bones and the heart with **calcium, magnesium, Vitamin D,** and **boron.** Go to your local health food store and ask for a supplement containing all four of these nutrients. If you take this supplement as directed before bedtime, the magnesium will lessen leg cramps and will promote a restful night's sleep.

- **Flaxseed oil** is a good source of omega-3 essential fatty acids, a nutrient necessary for the health of our cells. Research has suggested that flaxseed oil can also reduce the pain, inflammation, and swelling often associated with arthritis.

- I can't say enough about **glucosamine.** Glucosamine, with the nutrient **chondroitin,** does wonders for stiff joints. Take 1,500 mg of glucosamine and 1,200 mg of chondroitin daily to maintain healthy joint and connective tissue structure.

The above list of nutrients is just a small sample of the many minerals and vitamins necessary for our health as we age. Herbally speaking, the world of medicinal plants can also help keep us both physically and mentally fit. When using the following herbal remedies, take as directed on the label.

- The Greek hero Odysseus used **garlic** to protect himself from being turned into a pig. As mentioned earlier, this herb works wonders for naturally lowering cholesterol.

- The **gingko biloba** tree is believed to be the longest-living tree on Earth. No wonder this herb can effectively improve memory and thinking processes. Ginkgo also reduces inflammation.

  (**Note:** Do not use if you're on an anticoagulant medication or if you're going to be having a surgical procedure in the near future.)

- If you're a man over 40, don't forget the **saw palmetto.** This Native American herb has long been used as a "man's herb" because it's useful for the prostate and is thought to increase potency.

- Those pretty red berries growing in your hedge of **hawthorn** will strengthen the heart, lower high blood pressure, and regulate the heartbeat. (**Note:** Don't eat the berries.)

- Grab a good dose of vitamins with a cup of **nettle** tea. This herb is also used for arthritis and anemia.

- Once thought to help cure cataracts, **red clover** tea will not improve your vision, but it will assist your body in cleansing the blood.

- Help your liver do its job with an herbal remedy that's centuries old. Research has indicated that **milk thistle** seeds have a protective action on the liver.

- Get a boost of energy from a 7,000-year-old Chinese herb called **panax ginseng.** (**Note:** Do not use this herb if you have high blood pressure.)

If we're willing to take care of our nutritional needs, not only will we enjoy middle age, but we may live as long as my friend Mr. Harris. This chapter on aging is only meant to be a beginning. I hope you will take the time to continue exploring what you can do emotionally, physically, and spiritually to make this time in your life the best ever.

Eleanor took another sip of her herbal tea. "Yum. This is good. Kind of spicy. What is it?" she asked.

Smiling, I replied, "It's a common kitchen herb that has been found to have anti-aging properties."

Surprised, Eleanor asked, "Really? It must be one I'm not familiar with. How would I use this herb in my kitchen?"

Placing my own tea cup on the table, I answered, "Oh, let's see. You could use it on vegetables, with fish, and in gravies or spaghetti sauces."

Eleanor's eyes widened. "Okay," she said. "I give up. What is this secret anti-aging herb of yours?"

I then picked up a colorful box containing the tea bags and handed it to her.

Suddenly Eleanor burst out laughing. "Thyme? Regular thyme? That's incredible. You know, this aging thing just might turn out to be a lot of fun."

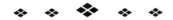

A*fterword*

THIS IS ONLY THE BEGINNING

In the preceding chapters, a wealth of healing suggestions for a number of specific mental health issues have been provided. Although numerous alternative health-care options have been presented, you, the reader, must understand that this book is only meant to be a beginning. That's it. A jump-start. My brief presentation of the many paths you can take to begin healing yourself is only the tip of the iceberg. There really is so much more to explore. A door has been opened for you, and you've walked into an exciting new world of self-care. Whether or not you continue this journey is up to you. I will tell you that once you've embarked on this path, it will be very hard to turn back. The sense of accomplishment that accompanies the experience of self-healing is very empowering. After such an experience, handing over total control of our health issues to health-care providers becomes very difficult, if not impossible.

After taking care of my alcohol and drug addiction, I needed to focus in on my Crohn's Disease. Once this illness was in remission, I had to address a food addiction. After I was nutritionally on track, my mental health program needed a little extra push. Taking control of my emotional, physical, and spiritual well-being required that I investigate everything from support groups to a variety of books on alternative healing methods. My Ph.D. in nutrition came as a direct result of my need to have more information on nutritional therapies. Next on my list of things to learn is acupuncture.

So, where will your travels take you? Leaving the pages of this book and moving on to other sources of self-healing is your next step. You may decide that you want to learn more about hypnotherapy, herbalism, nutrition, chiropractic care, Chinese medicine, Bach flower remedies, spiritual healing, or color therapy.

To help you with this "leap of faith," I have provided a list of resources you might want to explore. Find an alternative healing subject that really interests you. Read all you can on the topic. Look for classes that will help you further explore your new field of learning, and then incorporate this new philosophy of self-care into your life. After you've finished trekking down this particular road, move on to another.

Knowledge is a powerful tool, but with knowledge comes responsibility. I strongly believe that if you've read this far, you're ready to take on this task. My thoughts and prayers go with you as you embark on the road toward peak physical health, emotional well-being, and spiritual enlightenment.

Remember, *you* are your own best healer.

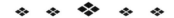

A*ppendix I*

HEALTHY BODY, WELL MIND DIET PLAN

A lthough we live in one of the most abundant societies in the world, many of us are subsisting on a diet that is nutritionally starving us. This starvation leads to numerous illnesses, both physical and emotional. To rectify this situation, here is a very simple diet plan to use as a foundation. Then build upon it with the suggestions from the chapter most suited to you.

Breakfast

In the book *Fit for Life,* by Harvey and Marilyn Diamond (1985), a simple breakfast solution is offered for the on-the-go person. Instead of that sweet roll or bagel with cream cheese, load up on fruits and vegetables. Is this such a far-fetched idea? No. In Israel, it's not uncommon to see salads as breakfast foods. Fruits have long been a breakfast food staple, especially in Europe. So, in the morning, eat as much fruit as you like. Grab some vegetable juice, an apple, and a banana as you're rushing out the door. Loaded with vitamins, fruits and veggies are easy to digest.

(**Note:** If you have a digestive disorder or have diabetes, talk to your health-care provider before implementing this breakfast plan.)

Lunch

This should be your biggest meal of the day, but keep it simple. We tend to overwork our digestive tracts by consuming too many different types of foods at once. If you choose to have protein, such as a meat or dairy product, for lunch, give your tummy a break by cutting out or down on the starches. Should you decide to have a starch for lunch, say a baked potato or a stir-fried rice dish, limit your protein intake. The standard American hamburger forces the digestive tract to work over-time. Be sure to pile on the vegetables. Your veggie intake for this meal should be three times that of your protein or starch dish. Finally, always keep sweets and fats to a minimum.

Dinner

With one exception, the rules for this meal are the same as above. The only difference between lunch and dinner is that your evening meal should be slightly smaller. Too much food too late in the evening will set off a fire alarm in your tummy at about 2:00 A.M.

(**Note:** If you're a vegetarian, separating starch from protein may not work for you. To make sure you're getting enough protein in your diet, combine grains with legumes.)

Snacks

Snacking is just fine *if* the foods you nibble on are not full of saturated fats, grease, and sugar. A little "pick-me-up" mid-morning, around 3 P.M., and just before bed, will keep blood sugar balanced and moodiness at bay. Exchange potato chips, cookies, candies, doughnuts, french fries, sugary sodas, and high-fat crackers with low-fat granola bars, fruits, whole grain breads, bits of dried fruit, a few almonds, herbal teas, fresh juices, or hearty rye crackers. Never snack on the run. Take time away from your busy day to sit, breathe, and enjoy the food you're eating.

Liquids

The human body needs 8–10 cups of water per day. Too many people in our culture think that liquid consumption consists of coffee, black tea, or soda pop. In my opinion, these liquids should not be considered to be part of the daily requirement for liquids. If your liquid consumption consists only of these beverages, you're at risk for dehydration and accompanying illnesses (such as kidney stones). Try to consume one glass of fresh fruit or vegetable juice; herbal tea; or clear, uncontaminated water every hour. Your body will thank you.

Remember: A healthy body is the foundation for natural mental health!

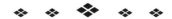

Appendix II

SUPPLEMENT FOR HEALTH

For years, there has been a great deal of controversy among physicians, nutritionists, and scientists in related fields over whether to supplement the diet with vitamin and mineral capsules or tablets. I strongly believe that a good all-purpose vitamin/mineral supplement is something that all of us should take daily. The American diet is deficient in many necessary nutrients. Because most American grains and produce are cultivated on farmland that is used year after year without organic supplementation, the nutrients in the soil are at risk for becoming depleted. In turn, this can leave the foods grown in such soil limited in nutritional value. For this reason alone, I urge all of my clients to take a trip to their local health food store and investigate the number of multivitamin/mineral supplements available on the market today.

Medical science, nutritionists, and most health-care workers know that vitamin and mineral deficiencies can lead to many physical and emotional illnesses. As a result, years ago, the federal government established guidelines to assist the population in determining whether their diets were deficient. The United States Food and Nutrition Board of the National Research Council has estimated the amount of nutrients we need to safeguard ourselves from extreme nutritional deficiency. The RDAs, or Recommended Daily Allowances, are periodically reevaluated and updated on a regular basis, but in 1985, this task became very complicated. Many of those involved in setting the RDA guidelines thought that the suggested nutrient dosages were too low for optimal health. Disagreement among the scientists involved in determining nutrient levels forced the National Research Council to delay releasing the new edition of guidelines until 1989.

Today, specific segments of the medical and scientific community continue to debate the RDA issue. These groups feel that the current RDA levels are not appropriate for optimal nutrition. Personally, I am in total agreement with these medical and scientific people. I strongly believe that the individual nutrient dosages, as listed in the RDA, are not high enough. Therefore, I'm going to list the RDAs for you with a definite purpose: to give you a vitamin/mineral foundation upon which you can build a nutrition program specifically for yourself. After reading the previous chapters and then reviewing those vitamin/mineral suggestions that best apply to you, use the RDA as a foundation upon which to build your initial supplementation program.

For example, according to the RDA, the adult woman or man only needs 60 mg of Vitamin C per day. In reviewing the chapter that fits your present situation, you may read that the suggested Vitamin C dose is 2,000 mg per day. If this is the case, you need to be ingesting the RDA's suggested dose of 60 mg of Vitamin C, along with 1,940 mg of additional Vitamin C. Take the suggested nutrient dose found in the chapter (in this case, it would be 2,000 mg), and subtract the RDA dose (which would be 60 mg in this example). This will give you the amount needed on top of the RDA suggested dose. (RDA—60 mg of Vitamin C, plus the added 1,940 mg of Vitamin C will give you the 2,000 mg dose suggested in the chapter that applies to you.) This is how you build your own personal vitamin/mineral profile.

If this seems like too much work for you, I suggest you get a copy of *Prescriptions for Nutritional Health,* by Balch and Balch (it's included in the reading list in the back of this book). Turn to page six of the Balchs' book, and you'll find a general vitamin/mineral profile with nutrient dosages that are higher than those presented in the RDA. Although these dosages are gauged for optimal nutritional health, remember that their suggested dosages are not a personalized profile.

I encourage you to develop your own profile before following Balchs', so let's look at the following list of RDAs. As I said earlier, use this chart as your guideline. Increase the dosages of each nutrient according to the nutritional suggestions in those chapters that apply to you. If you need help in doing so, seek out the assistance of a holistic nutritionist.

Supplement Daily Dosage

Vitamin A and Beta Carotene—Men: 5,000 IU; women: 4,000 IU

Vitamin D—Men and women: 200 IU

Vitamin E—Men: 15 IU; women: 12 IU

Vitamin K—Men: 80 mcg; women: 60 mcg

Vitamin F (essential fatty acids)—RDA is not identified

Vitamin B1, thiamin—Men: 1.5 mg; women: 1.1 mg

Vitamin B2, riboflavin—Men: 1.7 mg; women: 1.3 mg

Vitamin B3, niacin, nicotinamide—Men: 19 mg; women: 15mg

Vitamin B5, pantothenic Acid—Men: 4 mg; women: 7 mg

Vitamin B6, pyridoxine—Men: 2.0 mg; women: 1.6 mg

Biotin—Men and women: 0.3 mg

Folic acid, B9—Men: 0.2 mg; women: 0.18 mcg

Vitamin B12—Men and women: 2 mcg

Choline—Men and women: 100 mg

Inositol—Men and women: 100 mg

Vitamin B15, panagamic acid—RDA is not identified

Vitamin B17, amygdalin, nitrilosides—RDA is not identified

Vitamin C, ascorbic acid—Men and women: 60 mg

Vitamin P, bioflavonoids—RDA is not identified

Calcium—Men and women: 800 mg

Magnesium—Men: 350 mg; women: 280 mg

Potassium—Men and women: 2,000 mg

Sodium—Men and women: 500 mg

Phosphorus—Men and women: 800 mg

Chlorine—Men and women: 500 mg

Sulfur—RDA is not identified

Iron—Men: 10 mg; women: 15 mg

Iodine—Men and women: 150 mcg

Copper—Men and women: 1.5 to 3.0 mg

Zinc—Men and women: 15 mg

Silicon—RDA is not identified

Manganese—Men and women: 2.0 mg to 5.0 mg

Fluorine—RDA is not identified

Chromium—Men and women: 50 to 200 mcg Selenium—
Men: 70 mcg; women: 55 mcg

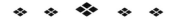

Self-help Resources

ADDICTION INFORMATION

Al-Anon, Al-Anon Adult Children of Alcoholics, and Al-Ateen Family Groups
P.O. Box 862
Midtown Station
New York, NY 10018

Alcohol and Drug Helpline
(800) 252-6465

Alcoholics Anonymous
475 Riverside Dr., 11th Floor
New York, NY 10015
(212) 870-6200

National Clearinghouse for Alcohol and Drug Information
11426–28 Rockville Pk., Ste. 200
Rockville, MD 20847-2345
(800) 729-6686

Pills Anonymous
P.O. Box 473
Ansonia Station
New York, NY 10023

AGING AND HEALTH

National Aging Information Center
500 E. Street, SW, Ste. 910
Washington, DC 20024-2710
(202) 554-9800

Alternative Healing Information and Resources
Acupressure Institute
1533 Shattuck Ave.
Berkeley, CA 94709
(800) 442-2232

American Aromatherapy Association
P.O. Box 606
San Rafael, CA 94915

American Herbal Association
P.O. Box 1673
Nevada City, CA 95959

American Holistic Health Association
P.O. Box 17400
Anaheim, CA 92817-7400
(714) 779-6152

American Holistic
Medicine Association
4101 Lake Boone Trail, Ste. 201
Raleigh, NC 27607

California School of
Herbal Studies
P.O. Box 39
Forestville, CA 95476

Herb Research
Foundation
1007 Pearl St., Ste. 200
Boulder, CO 80302
(303) 449-2265

Mind/Body Health
Sciences, Inc.
393 Dixon Rd.
Boulder, CO 80302
(303) 440-8460

BACH FLOWER REMEDIES

The Edward Bach Center
Sotwell Wallingford
Oxon OX10 OPZ
Great Britain
011-44-01-491-03-4678

CHILDREN

Attention Deficit
Disorder
Association
P.O. Box 972
Mentor, OH 44061
(800) 487-2282

CHINESE MEDICINE

American College of
Traditional
Chinese Medicine
455 Arkansas St.
San Francisco, CA 94107
(415) 282-7600

CHIROPRACTIC CARE

American Chiropractic
Association
1916 Wilson Blvd.
Arlington, VA 22201

FAMILY VIOLENCE
SUPPORT

Batterers Anonymous
P.O. Box 29
Redlands, CA 92373

Sexual Abuse
Anonymous
P.O. Box 80085
Minneapolis, MN 55408

Survivors Anonymous
18653 Ventura Blvd., Ste. 143
Tarzana, CA 91356

FOOD ALLERGY
RESOURCES

Feingold Association
of the United States
P.O. Box 6550
Alexandria, VA 22306
(703) 768-3287

Suggested Reading

Balch, James F., and Balch, Phyllis A. *Prescriptions for Nutritional Healing* (Second Edition). Avery Publishing Group, Garden City, New York, 1997.

Block, Marry Ann. *No More Ritalin.* Kensington Books, New York, 1996.

Chevallier, Andrew. *The Encyclopedia of Medicinal Plants.* Doring Kindersley, New York, 1996.

Cohen, Alan. *Happily Even After.* Hay House, Carlsbad, CA, 1999.

Collins, Terah Kathryn. *The Western Guide to Feng Shui— Room by Room.* Hay House, Carlsbad, CA, 1999.

Dean, Amy E. *Growing Older, Growing Better.* Hay House, Carlsbad, CA, 1997.

Diamond, Harvey and Diamond, Marilyn. *Fit for Life.* Warner Books, New York, 1985.

Guggenheim, Bill and Guggenheim, Judy. *Hello from Heaven.* Bantam Books, New York, 1997.

Hay, Louise L. *You Can Heal Your Life.* Hay House, Carlsbad, CA, 1984.

——. *Colors and Numbers.* Hay House, Carlsbad, CA, 1999.

Higley, Connie; Higley, Alan; and Leatham, Pat. *Aromatherapy A–Z.* Hay House, Carlsbad, CA, 1999.

Hoffman, David. *The Herbal Handbook: A User's Guide to Medical Herbalism.* Healing Arts Press, Rochester, Vermont, 1987.

Lerner, Harriet. *The Dance of Anger: A Woman's Guide to Changing the Patterns of Intimate Relationships.* Harper Collins, New York, 1997.

Jean-Murat, M.D., Carolle. *Menopause Made Easy.* Hay House, Carlsbad, CA, 1999.

Kroeger, Hanna. *Heal Your Life with Home Remedies and Herbs.* Hay House, Carlsbad, CA, 1998.

Lamb, Terry. *Born to Be Together.* Hay House, Carlsbad, CA, 1998.

Miller, Alice. *Thou Shalt Not Be Aware: Society's Betrayal of the Child.* NAL/Penguin, Inc., New York, 1986.

Plunckett, Jenny. *Traditional Herbal Remedies.* Paragon Book Services, Bristol, Great Britain, 1996.

Spiller, Gene and Hubbard, Rowena. *Nutritional Secrets of the Ancients.* Prima Publishing, Rocklin, CA, 1996.

Stengler, Angela and Stengler, Mark. *Natural Solutions for PMS: Top Herbal Remedies and More.* IMPAKT Communications, Inc., 1998.

Wills-Brandon, Carla. *Is It Love or Is It Sex? Why Relationships Don't Work.* Originally published by Health Communications, Inc, Deerfield Beach, Fl; 1989. Second printing: Back in Print, Shakespeare & Co. Booksellers, New York, 2000.

———. *Learning to Say No: Establishing Healthy Boundaries.* Originally published by Health Communications, Inc., Deerfield Beach, FL; 1990. Second printing: Back in Print, Shakespeare & Co. Booksellers, New York, 2000.

———. *One Last Hug Before I Go: Unlocking the Mystery Behind Death Bed Visions.* Health Communications, Inc., Deerfield Beach, FL, 2000.

Young, Jacqueline. *Acupressure: Step by Step—the Oriental Way to Health.* Thorsons Publishing, 1998.

About the Author

Carla Wills-Brandon has a Ph.D. in nutrition and is the author of six previously published books, five of which were for Health Communications, Inc. She works as a Licensed Marriage and Family Therapist with her child psychologist husband, Michael Brandon. The Brandons have their private practice in a 100-year-old house just outside of Houston, Texas. Dr. Wills-Brandon specializes in trauma resolution, spiritual well-being, and grief.

Dr. Wills-Brandon has lectured across the United States and in the United Kingdom. Also, she has made guest appearances on *Geraldo, Montel, Sally Jessy Raphael, The Marilu Henner Show, The Faith Daniels Show,* and numerous other television and radio programs.

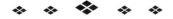

Other Hay House
Titles of Related Interest

Aromatherapy 101, by Karen Downes

*Constant Craving: What Your Food Cravings
Mean and How to Overcome Them,*
by Doreen Virtue, Ph.D.

Deep Healing: The Essence of Mind/Body Medicine,
by Emmett Miller, M.D.

*The Essential Flower Essence Handbook:
Remedies for Inner Well-Being,* by Lila Devi

Heal Your Body A–Z, by Louise L. Hay

The Indigo Children: The New Kids Have Arrived,
by Lee Carroll and Jan Tober

Heal Your Life with Home Remedies and Herbs,
by Hanna Kroeger

Natural Pregnancy A–Z, by Carolle Jean-Murat, M.D.

*Reclaiming Goddess Sexuality:
The Power of the Feminine Way,*
by Linda Savage, Ph.D.

The Steps to Healing, by Dana Ullman, M.P.H.

*Whose Face Is in the Mirror:
The Story of One Woman's Journey from the
Nightmare of Domestic Abuse to True Healing,*
by Dianne Schwartz

Your Personality, Your Health, by Carol Ritberger, Ph.D.

All of the above titles
can be ordered through your local bookstore, or
by calling Hay House at (800) 654-5126.